understanding
DIABETES

by JOHN W. STEPHENS, M.D.

THE TOUCHSTONE PRESS
P. O. Box 81
Beaverton, Oregon 97005

understanding
DIABETES

A reference book about adult-onset diabetes and about juvenile diabetes, emphasizing the peculiarities of each and their treatment.

Other areas receiving special attention are hypoglycemia in the diabetic, hyperlipidemia, obesity, pregnancy, travel and adjustment to time zone changes.

A Section With Diabetic Recipes Is Included

By John W. Stephens, M.D.
Clinical Professor of Medicine, University of Oregon Medical School;
Physician, Good Samaritan Hospital and Medical Center,
Portland, Oregon.

And Otto C. Page, M.D.
Associate Clinical Professor of Medicine, University of Oregon Medical School; Physician, Good Samaritan Hospital and Medical Center.
Robert L. Hare, M.D.
Professor of Medicine, University of Oregon Medical School; Physician, Good Samaritan Hospital and Medical Center.
Liz Burke, R.N.
Coordinator Diabetes Education Program, Good Samaritan Hospital and Medical Center, Portland, Oregon.

— CONTENTS —

PART 1   NATURE of DIABETES — General comments 8
         CHAPTER 1 — ADULT ONSET DM 17
         CHAPTER 2 — JUVENILE DIABETES 27

PART 2   DIETARY MANAGEMENT — General comments 36
         CHAPTER 3 — THE CALCULATED DIET 46
         CHAPTER 4 — THE EXCHANGE DIET 67
         CHAPTER 5 — OTHER DIET INFORMATION 76

PART 3   CHAPTER 6 — ORAL TREATMENT OF DM 82
         CHAPTER 7 — INSULIN TREATMENT OF DM 84
         CHAPTER 8 — HYPOGLYCEMIA 100
         CHAPTER 9 — URINE TESTING 108
         CHAPTER 10 — TREATMENT DURING ILLNESS .. 115
         CHAPTER 11 — FOOT CARE 120

PART 4   CHAPTER 12 — COMPLICATIONS OF DM:
                      — DIABETIC KETOACIDOSIS 124
                      — DIABETIC NEURITIS 126
                      — ATHEROSCLEROSIS 127
                      — DISORDERS OF KIDNEY
                        FUNCTION 127
                      — DISORDERS OF VISION 128

PART 5   OTHER ASPECTS OF LIVING WITH DIABETES:
         CHAPTER 13 — OBESITY — HYPERLIPIDEMIA ... 134
         CHAPTER 14 — MENSTRUATION — PREGNANCY . 139
         CHAPTER 15 — EMPLOYABILITY and INSURANCE 143
         CHAPTER 16 — TRAVEL SUGGESTIONS 146

PART 6   RECIPES FOR THE DIABETIC 152

PART 7   APPENDIX   — RESOURCE LISTS 180
                    — GLOSSARY 183
         ALPHABETICAL INDEX 188

Introduction

The physician who treats patients with diabetes mellitus assumes a number of responsibilities and has to accept challenges which reach beyond those relating to the immediate complaint of the patient. Following the diagnosis and institution of appropriate treatment, he must help the patient prepare to fulfill family and employment obligations, to attain educational and other ambitions, to bear children, enjoy leisure hours; in summary, to lead a full life. As Dr. M. G. Candaw, Director General of the World Health Organization, stated in his World Health Day message on April 7, 1971: "Obviously, certain precautions must be taken. The most important is that the treatment and dietary regime prescribed by the doctor are carefully followed. Diabetic patients must also subject themselves to a periodical 'check-up'. This is particularly true during or after an illness such as influenza, or during pregnancy. For people about to be married, genetic counseling is advisable when either partner has a family history of diabetes." He goes on to report that "the more people know about the disease the better they will be able to fight it."

The patient, in turn, should be aware of the fact that with so many concerns for a chronic illness, the physician may not be totally effective in dealing with every aspect of the disease. The physician is trained to assess the complaints of a patient with the assistance of appropriate physical and laboratory examinations. A successful encounter during an acute illness results in a well and happy patient and a physician rewarded by the knowledge that his patient is once again healthy and content. When the physician prepares to help a patient with a chronic disease, however, there is attention not only to the immediate needs of the patient, but preparations are initiated for continuing care: i.e., with the assistance of other health professionals, education to understand the disease and the total implications of neglect in relation to future health, budget, employment, and so forth. Above all there is a need to persuade or motivate the person with diabetes to develop the capacity and desire to successfully manage his illness. **In this way both the patient and the physician having shared the responsibility of treatment, may together enjoy the rewards of accomplishment.** However, if either feels a lack of interest or sees inadequate effort on the part of the other, there will be a loss of enthusiasm, and a less effective relationship.

Now to the business at hand, diabetes mellitus (D.M.) and, in particular, assistance to those who desire guidance and are willing to cooperate in its management. . . .

PREFACE

This manual is designed to serve as a reference book for persons with diabetes, their family members, and for nurses and dietitians interested in training of those who have been referred for education and treatment.

Persons with abnormally elevated blood sugar levels usually have one of two forms of diabetes mellitus. However, there are other causes of abnormally elevated blood sugar levels: e.g., hyperlipidemias, which require special dietary measures. Therefore we have concluded it is best to center individual instruction on the type of diabetes or other disease present. For this reason the book is divided into sections. It is recommended that readers initially limit their reading to those sections which are most applicable to their situation.

The majority of persons with diabetes mellitus have the adult-onset stable form of diabetes. Chapter 1 discusses this variety of diabetes mellitus, which can occur at any age, but most often occurs after the age of 40. This form is characterized by freedom from, or only mild symptoms of diabetes, modest elevations of blood glucose (sugar), and the probability of considerable improvement by achievement of normal weight by dietary measures.

Chapter 2 deals with the more acute form of diabetes. It is characterized by the presence of signs and symptoms due to lack of insulin, and an elevated blood sugar, sometimes complicated by the presence of ketones. This form of diabetes is most common in juveniles but also occurs in a small percentage of adults. The treatment must be more aggressive, utilizing not only certain dietary recommendations but the use of insulin. Often the adult patient achieves improved control by using one of the oral agents in conjunction with a prescribed diet. Individuals with this type of diabetes are more sensitive to external stresses such as infections and, for this reason, must be able to recognize those factors which can aggravate or change the control of their diabetes so that they might quickly institute corrective procedures. These factors will be discussed.

A third group is composed of persons who have what is called a disorder of lipoprotein metabolism. Usually, these persons are young-to-middle-aged individuals who are overweight. They may have initially received information that their blood serum was milky after being allowed to stand, or that their blood cholesterol is high. The milky serum reflects the presence of a large amount of triglycerides (a type of fat) in the blood. Failure to correct the situation leads to characteristic skin, vascular and metabolic changes. This pattern of events can be altered by careful restriction of calories and in some the intake of carbohydrate foods. This step overcomes the special metabolic defect, which is one of abnormal conversion of carbohydrate into excessive amounts of triglycerides. Others must restrict foods contributing to elevation of the blood cholesterol. Hyperlipidemia is reviewed in Chapter 13.

More and more, we recognize that some people with excess weight have more than just the problem of simply overeating. They may also have certain disorders of metabolism, permitting the body to form and maintain fat deposits, leading to an overweight condition. Many seek help for weight control, not only because of the inconvenience of excess weight, but because of the increased health hazards. Therefore, we have introduced a section on obesity to assist people with this problem.

We are indebted to many persons. We must specifically thank those from whom we have learned, in particular those with diabetes, those with whom we have worked and those who have stimulated us to produce this book.

Deserving special thanks for helping in the preparation of the book are Ms. Marjorie Yung, and Ms. Mary Laird, former or present instructors in our teaching program at Good Samaritan Hospital and Medical Center; Dr. John Galloway, Medical Director, Eli Lilly and Company, Indianapolis, Indiana, who reviewed the material and offered significant suggestions; and Ms. Jean Roberts for her valued secretarial assistance.

The manuscript was read and edited by my daughter, Ruth Ann Dodson, and by Thomas K. Worcester, The Touchstone Press. This generous contribution of time and skill is greatly appreciated. Also much appreciated was the assistance of Oral Bullard, Publisher, The Touchstone Press.

J.W.S.

Portland, Oregon
January, 1975

Part 1

THE NATURE OF DIABETES MELLITUS

THE NATURE OF DIABETES MELLITUS
— General Comments —

Diabetes may seem a calamity to someone newly introduced to the condition. But to those educated and experienced in its management, diabetes is nothing more than a nuisance. Converting diabetes from calamity to nuisance requires a measure of time, a small but important store of knowledge, and an open mind.

Diabetes mellitus* (D.M.) is a medical term used to describe a condition in which the body tissues are unable to utilize or store glucose (sugar) normally. As a result, greater than normal amounts of unused glucose are found in the bloodstream and some body tissues. Eventually, the level of blood glucose becomes sufficiently high to cause the kidneys to lose glucose in the urine. The diagnosis of D.M. is dependent on these findings. For a clear understanding of the nature of D.M. it is helpful to review where glucose comes from and how it is used in the normal state.

WHERE DOES BLOOD GLUCOSE COME FROM?

Glucose always is present in the bloodstream. It is essential for body energy and is available constantly either from digestion of food or from conversion of body stores.

When carbohydrate foods — foods containing sugars and starches — are eaten, they are broken down into simple sugar molecules by digestive juices. In a liquid state, these molecules enter the bloodstream through tiny blood vessels in the walls of the small intestine. (Fig. 1)

During short periods of fasting, glucose is made available to the body by the liver which may either release stored glucose taken previously from the bloodstream, or may release glucose manufactured by the liver from body protein. Thus the body is assured of a ready supply of blood sugar.

WHERE DOES BLOOD GLUCOSE GO?

The blood vessels in the body make up a vast pipeline which transports a variety of essential substances to every body cell and carries away

*Aretaeus the Cappadocian, living during the time of the Roman Empire, is reported to be the first to use the word diabetes.

waste products. Glucose moving through the bloodstream is picked up and used by many body tissues, primarily in these four areas:

1. Muscle cells: to provide energy for muscle work.
2. Liver cells: to store it as glycogen for later use; convert excess glucose to triglyceride.
3. Brain and Nerve cells: to give energy.
4. Fat cells: to store surplus glucose (which has been converted in the liver, to triglyceride) as adipose fat.

The ability of muscle, liver and fat cells to use glucose when it reaches its destination, depends upon the action of insulin. Only brain cells appear to make use of glucose without insulin.

WHAT IS INSULIN?

Insulin is a protein substance produced in specialized cells clustered within the pancreas (Islets of Langerhans). Insulin is released into the bloodstream by these cells (Beta cells) when they are stimulated by an elevation of blood glucose levels.

Insulin may be thought of as a chemical key that unlocks the doors of cells allowing glucose to enter. In the presence of adequate insulin, the cell bodies remove glucose from the bloodstream and prevent the blood glucose level from becoming excessive. (Fig. 1)

NORMAL BLOOD GLUCOSE LEVELS

With adequate insulin, blood glucose levels fluctuate within a relatively narrow range. The following levels are recognized as normal:

TIME IN RELATION TO MEAL	NORMAL GLUCOSE VALUES BLOOD	PLASMA
FASTING	60-120 mg.	70-140 mg.
1 Hour*	Less than 160 mg.	Less than 185 mg.
2 Hours*	Less than 120 mg.	Less than 140 mg.

*Following High Carbohydrate Meal or a Glucose Load.

These normal levels result from a delicate balance between insulin production and storage or release of glucose by the liver. Plasma or serum glucose values are 15 percent higher than blood glucose values. After age 45, plasma glucuse values may be higher by 10 mg. per decade at one hour and maybe 4 to 6 mg. at two hours after intake of glucose.

When the blood glucose level begins to rise, insulin is released from the pancreas and aids the transfer of glucose into cells. This prevents a rise beyond normal values. When the glucose level value falls too low, insulin production diminishes. The liver releases its stored sugar, thus preventing the blood glucose level from becoming too low.

RESULTS OF TOO LITTLE INSULIN

When the insulin-producing cells fail to respond adequately to a rise in blood glucose the following events occur:

1. Blood glucose rises to higher than normal levels. Initially, the disorder of insulin secretion is slight, so that abnormal elevations in blood glucose may only appear after high carbohydrate intake. There is still sufficient insulin to correct the elevated blood glucose values. With more severe insulin deficiency, the blood glucose may be elevated at all times. (Fig. 2)

2. Glucose appears in the urine when the blood values for glucose rise sufficiently to exceed the "spilling point" at which the kidneys are no longer able to conserve glucose. The blood level at which glucose is lost through the kidneys is usually 160 mg. per 100 ml. (but often exceeds 200 mg. in older people). When only small amounts of glucose are lost in the urine there are no problems. However, as larger amounts appear the following symptoms may occur:

  A. Frequent and copious urination: increased sugar carried out in the urine results in a larger amount of urine formed.
  B. Increasing thirst and sense of dryness caused by the passage of large amounts of urine.
  C. Weight loss occurring when the combined loss of glucose in the urine and calories converted to energy by the body exceed those contributed by intake of food.

3. The liver begins to produce sugar from body protein. Normally, this occurs during fasting or times of unusual stress, but it also occurs abnormally in uncontrolled diabetes.

WHEN DOES D.M. DEVELOP AND WHY?

Although diabetes has been recognized for more than a thousand years, its basic cause remains unknown. It is discovered more often in individuals over the age of 45 years, but is not necessarily a disease of old age. In the United States more females than males have diabetes. Nearly six out of seven of those developing diabetes after the age of 45 are overweight.

INHERITANCE: Since the classical studies of Drs. Pincus and White[1]

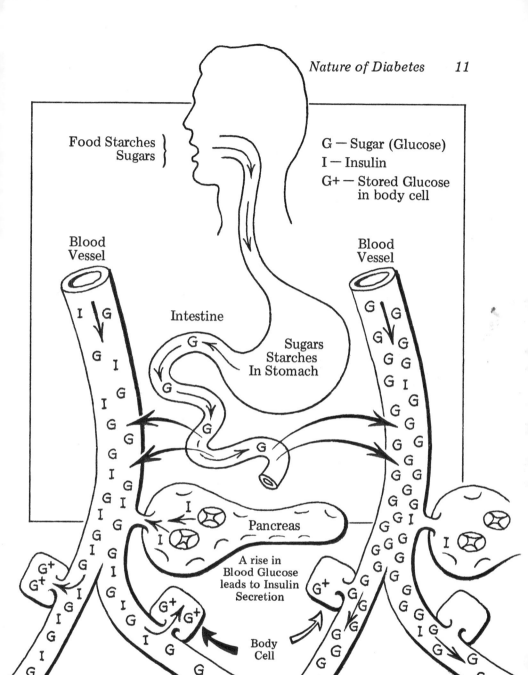

FIG. 1 — The effect of ingestion of carbohydrate foods on the concentration of blood glucose (G), insulin production (I), and the effect of insulin on glucose entry into body cells (G+).

FIG. 2 — The effect of ingestion of carbohydrate foods and lack of insulin release on the level of blood glucose (G) which is accompanied by a decrease in uptake of (G+) by body cells.

CONCEPT OF RECESSIVE HEREDITY AND
PROBABILITY OF INDIVIDUAL DEVELOPING D.M.

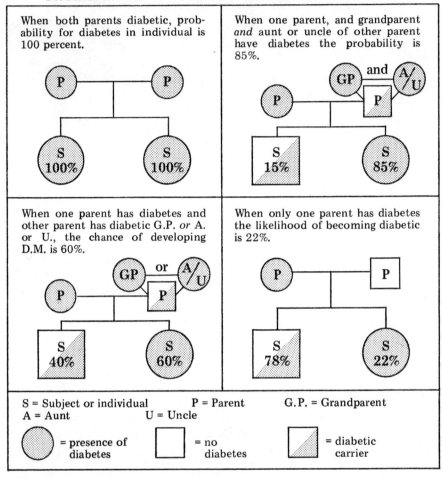

When both parents diabetic, probability for diabetes in individual is 100 percent.

When one parent, and grandparent *and* aunt or uncle of other parent have diabetes the probability is 85%.

When one parent has diabetes and other parent has diabetic G.P. *or* A. or U., the chance of developing D.M. is 60%.

When only one parent has diabetes the likelihood of becoming diabetic is 22%.

S = Subject or individual   P = Parent   G.P. = Grandparent
A = Aunt   U = Uncle

= presence of diabetes   = no diabetes   = diabetic carrier

FIG. 3 — When there is a family history of diabetes, tests of other family members are indicated under the following circumstances.

1. Symptoms of diabetes
2. Obesity
3. Coronary heart disease
4. Mothers with obstetrical history of:
   a. Large babies (particularly increasing birth weight with each succeeding pregnancy).
   b. Miscarriages or stillbirths.
   c. Excessive fluid retention during pregnancy.

demonstrated a significant familial incidence of D.M., the concept of recessive inheritance of diabetes has been accepted. On this assumption it is possible to indicate a theoretical inheritance pattern for diabetes. (Fig. 3) However, the variable age of onset and the variations in severity of the disease make genetical analysis difficult. Dr. Nancy Simpson[2] of Toronto, Canada, reported after a study of juvenile diabetics that a simple mode of inheritance could not always be applied and that "multifactorial inheritance" (a number of inherited factors) is a more reasonable basis from which to study inheritance. Insulin cell function, endocrine gland activity (e.g., excess glucagon production), insulin antagonism, and obesity are all factors which relate to specific genetic action. That obesity and inheritance of diabetes interact has been demonstrated by Dr. J. D. Baird[3] of Great Britain. His study found that while diabetes was three times as common in siblings of diabetic persons, the rate was highest in the obese siblings of non-obese diabetics.

Dr. J. E. Craighead and his co-workers[4] at the University of Vermont have produced diabetes in mice by injection of the encephalomyocarditis viruses. These viruses attack the pancreas of the test animals. Dr. D. R. Gamble and colleagues[5] in England have reported that juvenile diabetes occurs more frequently in the fall and winter, at a time when there is a greater incidence of certain virus infections. This interest in viruses as a potential cause of diabetes has led Drs. H. L. Levy and A. L. Notkins to suggest that certain persons, by being genetically predisposed, would thereby inherit a susceptibility to viral causes of diabetes. This would occur because the special receptor sites on the beta cells (insulin source cells) that regulate insulin secretion would be susceptible to the effects of the viruses. It is not possible to draw any conclusions at this time about the role of viruses in causing diabetes. Interest at this time centers on rubella, mumps, and coxsackie B viruses.

INHERITED DIABETES: ITS RELATIONSHIP TO ALPHA AND BETA CELL FUNCTION

It is well established that inherited diabetes is related to disordered function of the pancreas beta cells resulting in lack of insulin. In 1970, Dr. Roger Unger and associates[6] in Dallas reported that there is also an excess of glucagon in the blood. Glucagon is a secretion of the alpha cells of the pancreas. Normally, elevation of the blood glucagon level occurs in association with low blood glucose levels (HYPO-GLYCEMIA). It is inappropriate, therefore, to find elevation of blood glucagon where there is an elevation of blood glucose. This suggests that persons with inherited diabetes have two malfunctions — failure of the beta cell function and overactivity of the alpha cells, possibly a bi-hormonal disease. This is considered to be a most important observation. In 1972, Dr. Roger Guillemin and his colleagues[7] identified a substance, somatostatin, which is described more fully in the section on diabetic retinopathy, Chapter 12. Dr. C. H. Mortimer and his associates[8] in Britain, and other investigators in Denmark and Britain have shown that somatostatin impairs the release not only of insulin, but also of glucagon. Applying this information, Dr. Peter Forsham and his fellow researchers in San Francisco have studied the role of soma-tostatin in the treatment of diabetic patients. By suppressing the elevated blood levels of glucagon, the blood glucose levels are suppressed significantly. They anticipate that the use of somatostatin with insulin will greatly ease the management and control of diabetes.

INCIDENCE

The American Diabetes Association (A.D.A.) reports that there are over four million in the United States with D.M., and one third of them are unaware of it. The Joslin Clinic reports that one woman in fifty and one man in one hundred in the 55 to 65 age group have D.M. About one in 2000 children have it.

PRECIPITATING FACTORS: While the onset of diabetes may not be associated with any unusual happening or change in general health status, there are several known conditions or factors which may precede D.M. in those who have inherited the tendency.

1. Obesity
Adult diabetes occurs more frequently in those who are significantly overweight. In fact, Dr. Kelly West and his associates[9], of Oklahoma City, have produced evidence that obesity is **the** most important of the environmental factors contributing to adult onset diabetes. The reason for this is not clear. It may be the result of increased insulin production causing obesity or vice-versa (See p. 20). Many obese persons are less sensitive to the effects of insulin. In a significantly high percentage of cases the blood glucose values return to normal after some weight loss.

2. Stress
Frequently the signs and symptoms of diabetes become apparent during or immediately after a period of significant stress, examples of which are:
    A. Acute illness, e.g. infection
    B. Surgery or serious accident

C. Emotional stress

D. Pregnancy

3. Use of certain medications:
   A. Cortisone, epinephrine
   B. Oral contraceptives — though these are not considered a cause of D.M.
   C. Certain diuretics, e.g. thiazides
   D. Nicotinic acid (high dose use over long period of time)

NON-INHERITED FORMS OF D.M.

These occur infrequently and are the result of:

1. Direct destruction of the insulin producing cells by certain diseases of the pancreas.

2. Interference with insulin secretion and/or overproduction of blood glucose, e.g. epinephrine-producing adrenal tumor, overproduction of blood glucose, e.g. cortisone-producing adrenal tumor.

3. Interference with action of insulin — growth hormone from pituitary tumor.

CAN D.M. BE PREVENTED?

We do not yet know enough about diabetes mellitus to give solid recommendations for its prevention. In the meantime, individuals with a family history of diabetes should recognize that diabetes is more likely to occur among the offspring of two parents with a family history of diabetes. The incidence is also higher than normal when one parent has diabetes. It is also important for persons with a family history of diabetes to avoid being overweight. Obesity is associated with excessive demands upon the insulin-secreting cells. Correction of obesity results in a decrease in insulin secretion and thereby helps to preserve the function of the insulin-producing cells. Decreased consumption of sweets is suggested for those who are overweight and who need to restrict caloric intake.

THOUGHTS ABOUT THE TREATMENT OF D.M.

Some difference of opinion exists among physicians concerning the objectives of treatment of D.M. On the other hand, there are some areas of complete agreement.

1. ALL PHYSICIANS AGREE THAT TREATMENT SHOULD:
   A. Prevent diabetic ketoacidosis and serious hypoglycemia.
   B. Be directed toward good control of diabetes co-existing with

pregnancy.

C. Control diabetes sufficiently to correct and prevent signs and symptoms of diabetes.

D. Encourage correction of excessive weight.

2. SOME PHYSICIANS, INCLUDING THE AUTHORS, FURTHER STRESS THAT TREATMENT SHOULD:

A. Be of a degree that will:

   1) Improve resistance to infections, particularly of the kidneys and urinary bladder.

   2) Decrease the frequency of diabetic neuritis (See page 126).

   3) Possibly delay the appearance of serious degenerative changes in blood vessels.

B. Be adjusted according to the needs and aspirations of the diabetic person. There are occasions when careful individualization of treatment measures* must be made.

C. Help to strengthen and encourage the patient with diabetes, to alleviate his anxieties while at the same time helping him understand the nature of his disease.

---

*The treatment measures will not be discussed at this point but will be covered in the sections which follow in relation to what is desired and achievable for each group of diabetic patients.

[1] Pincus, G., and White, P. (1933) On the Inheritance of Diabetes Mellitus, 1. An Analysis of 675 Family Histories. *Amer. Jour. of Med. Sc.,* 186:1.

[2] Simpson, N. (1964) Multifactorial Inheritance: A Possible Hypothesis for Diabetes. *Diabetes* 13:462.

[3] Baird, J. D., et al. (1967) Medical and Scientific Section of the British Diabetic Association.

[4] Craighead, J. E. (1972) Workshop on Viral Infection and Diabetes Mellitus in Man. National Institutes of Health. *Jour. Infect. Diseases* 125:568.

[5] Gamble, D. R., et al. (1969) Viral Antibodies in Diabetes Mellitus. *British Med. Jour.* 3:627.

[6] Unger, R. H., et al. (1970) Studies of Pancreatic Alpha Cell Function in Normal and Diabetic Subjects. *Jour. Clin. Investig.* 49:837.

[7] Brazeau, P., et al. (1973) Hypothalmic Polypeptide that Inhibits the Secretion of Immunoreactive Pituitary Growth Hormone. *Science, N.Y.* 179:77.

[8] Mortimer, C. H., et al. (1974) Effects of Growth-Hormone Release-Inhibiting Hormone on Circulating Glucagon, Insulin and Growth Hormone in Normal, Diabetic, Acromegalic and Hypopituitary Patients. *The Lancet.* 1:697.

[9] West, K. M., et al. (1971) Influences of Nutritional Factors on Prevalence of Diabetes. *Diabetes* 20:99.

Chapter 1 ADULT ONSET DIABETES MELLITUS

ADULT ONSET DIABETES MELLITUS

This chapter of the book is directed to those who developed diabetes mellitus in their adult years. It discusses characteristics that are unique to the adult onset type of D.M. References are made to other sections of the book for information concerning the management and treatment of some additional problems related to adult onset diabetes.

WHAT DISTINGUISHES ADULT ONSET DIABETES MELLITUS?

Adult diabetes mellitus (D.M.) is one of the two principal types of diabetes. It is most frequently discovered in individuals over 45 years of age. As the onset is slow and often without readily recognized symptoms, it may come to light only during a routine physical examination. On occasion itchiness of the skin, an infection of the foot, loss of sensation for heat or pain in the feet, or blurred vision may have led to a visit to the physician.

□‡ *SYMPTOMS OF ADULT ONSET DIABETES*

Infections — skin or urinary tract   Decreased pain and heat sensation
Foot — ulcers, corns, callouses   in the feet
Dry, itchy skin   Blurred vision

This form of D.M. has certain features that distinguish it from the juvenile type: 1) Eighty percent of these adults are overweight. 2) In 1968 Dr. Glen McDonald, then Chief of the Diabetes and Arthritis Control Program, National Center for Chronic Disease Control,* reported survey results indicating that although 84 percent reported no severe disability due to diabetes, other conditions caused some disability in 58 percent of those interviewed (heart conditions, high blood pressure, impaired vision). 3) Acute symptoms of D.M. (to be discussed under Juvenile Diabetes) are infrequent, as is the condition known as ketoacidosis. Most adult individuals feel perfectly healthy until some complication or other illness develops.

*Characteristics of Persons with Diabetes, United States — July 1964 — June 1965. Natl. Center for Health Statistics Series 10, No. 40. Washington, D.C.: Gov't Printing Office, 1967.

‡ □ designates highlights or summary of subject reviewed.

□ CHARACTERISTICS OF ADULT ONSET DIABETES

Onset — gradual
Symptoms — May be absent — Rarely acute as in juvenile
Overweight — 70-80% of cases
Ketoacidosis — rare
Treatment* — Diet alone — 25% — With insulin — 25% (until recently)
— With oral RX — 50%

There is considerable interest in the reasons for differences between adult and juvenile forms of D.M. — both of which can occur in the same families. One finding that sheds some light on this difference, first described by Drs. Yalow and Berson[1], relates to the level of insulin normally found in the blood during an oral glucose (sugar) tolerance test. The individual with adult onset diabetes is not only capable of secreting insulin from the pancreas, but the obese adult diabetic often secretes an amount **greater** than that secreted by a non-diabetic person. The problem is that the insulin is more slowly released. (Fig. 4) Dr. D. Kipnis[2] of St. Louis has demonstrated that diabetic children fail to secrete insulin in response to oral glucose testing.

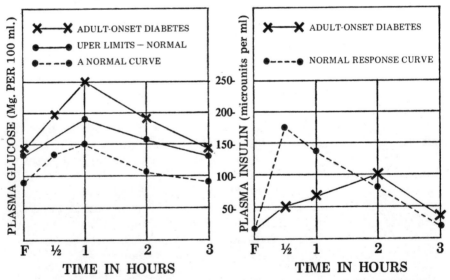

Fig. 4 — Plasma glucose and plasma insulin responses to an oral glucose tolerance test in adult-onset diabetes. (F=fasting)

*Characteristics of Persons with Diabetes, United States — July 1964 — June 1965. Natl. Center for Health Statistics Series 10, No. 40. Washington, D.C.: Gov't Printing Office, 1967.

Since most individuals with adult onset diabetes secrete insulin in relation to eating, utilization of carbohydrate in the body continues. This prevents the blood glucose from rising so high that symptoms of diabetes develop.

WHY TREAT THIS FORM OF D.M.?

Earlier it was pointed out that many with this form of D.M. feel quite well and are even surprised to discover that they have diabetes. It is difficult to generate enthusiasm for a disease that seems neither severe nor disruptive. Why then must one accept treatment? The reasons are directed to two aspects of the problem. An additional benefit can relate to employability.

1. *OBESITY* — often is associated with this type of D.M. and is itself considered a health hazard. Overweight individuals are subject to such health problems as: possibly coronary (heart) artery disease; hypertension (high blood pressure); cerebral artery disease causing strokes; gall bladder disease; degenerative arthritis, particularly of the knees and hips; respiratory problems causing shortness of breath; hernias; and socioeconomic related problems leading to emotional stresses.*

☐ *OBESITY RELATED HEALTH HAZARDS*

    Coronary artery disease
    Cerebral artery disease
    High blood pressure
    Gall bladder disease
    Arthritis
    Hernias
    Respiratory insufficiency
    Emotional strain

2. *DIABETES* — though often mild in association with excess weight, may later cause complications. Some of these are aggravated by being overweight, e.g. hardening of the arteries leading to heart problems, strokes, lack of circulation in the feet; a form of neuritis which may lead to loss of appreciation for heat and pain in the legs; ulcers of the feet; impairment of vision due to damaged blood vessels. These diseases may lead to considerable disability and impairment of health as well as reduce longevity.

*Edit. THE LANCET 1:381-2, Feb. 20, 1971.

□ *CONDITIONS OCCURRING IN ASSOCIATION WITH ADULT ON-SET DIABETES MELLITUS*

Arteriosclerosis (thickening of the arteries) affecting:

Heart
Brain
Kidneys
Legs

Neuritis
Damage to blood vessels — eyes
Foot ulcers

3. *EMPLOYABILITY* — is improved for those whose diabetes is controlled by diet. For example, there is less difficulty acquiring a private pilot's license, a chauffeur's license, or qualifying as a railroad engineer (See also p. 143).

OBJECTIVES OF TREATMENT

1. *WEIGHT REDUCTION* — Excessive weight is associated with an enlarging of body fat cells. These enlarged cells attract or require increasing amounts of insulin — causing a drain on the insulin producing cells. This can be overcome by weight reduction which in turn leads to a decrease in the severity of this form of diabetes.

2. *REDUCTION IN SEVERITY AND COMPLICATIONS OF D.M.* — milder diabetes, as indicated above, results from weight reduction. This is considered helpful in preventing certain complications of diabetes. Dr. M.D. Siperstein[3] of San Francisco, California, has suggested, as a result of his investigations of the thickness of the inner layer of muscle capillaries (small blood vessels), that many persons with diabetes have not only inherited this disease but also a tendency toward small blood vessel disease. Dr. J. R. Williamson and his co-workers[4] in St. Louis, Mo., after similar studies of the thickness of muscle capillary basement membrane thickening (BMT) concluded, "The incidence and magnitude of BMT increase with longer known duration of diabetes." Furthermore, they concluded that BMT is probably normal prior to the onset of diabetes. BMT is seen as a consequence of aging in both normals and diabetics. Many physicians consider this process to be furthered by poorly controlled diabetes. Dr. R. A. Guthrie has found this to be so in children. He reported that children with well controlled diabetes were free of unusual BMT after diabetes of 15 years duration, whereas poorly controlled children showed significant thickening within a period of five years.*

*First International Workshop on Diabetes and Camping. Editors Etzwiler D. D. and Robb, J. R.

□ *OBJECTIVES IN TREATMENT OF ADULT ONSET D.M.*

Produce milder form of D.M.
Reduce body weight
Decrease incidence of complications of:
  a. Diabetes
  b. Obesity
Improved sense of well-being
Improved life expectancy

TREATMENT OF ADULT ONSET D.M.

Treatment in most cases is directed at weight reduction and reducing the blood glucose level to a normal range. This is achieved by a DIET restricting calorie intake. For a smaller number it may mean the addition of insulin or possibly the use of one of the oral diabetic tablets. Of nearly equal importance is a program of regular exercise.

DIET

The diet low in calories for those who are overweight will also be necessarily low in fat and carbohydrate foods. This restriction is continued until sufficient weight loss has occurred. The meal plan can permit three or more meals a day. Low-calorie dietary supplements are helpful and contribute to the acceptability of a low-calorie diet. Occasionally people look for other means to help them reach their desired weight more rapidly. As a result, they are susceptible to exploitation by some commercial organizations. No drug is yet available that will safely and effectively control the appetite. Some groups, operating along the lines similar to Alcoholics Anonymous, may, by offering moral support and encouragement, increase the chances of adhering to a restricted dietary program.

The principles of diet construction and menu planning are covered in Part 2.

EXERCISE on a regular basis improves health prospects even for the perfectly healthy. Energy is expended during exercise. Our carbohydrate and fat foods are sources of energy. If these are restricted in the diet, energy for exercise may be supplied by body stores of fat and sugar. Whether exercise aids in any significant way to weight loss depends upon the amount and duration of time involved. (See Table I.) A 150 pound man expends 150-400 calories per hour above the basal or resting level while walking. Walking still remains the most readily available and inexpensive form of exercise. Such activity helps to regulate obesity and improve muscle tone. It also contributes significantly to improved oxygen utilization by the heart and circulation in the arteries of the heart and legs, not to mention one's increased sense of vitality.

TABLE 1 — GROSS EXPENDITURE OF ENERGY
Mean Values Expressed in Calories

	BODY WEIGHT (pounds)	CALORIES per hour
Sleeping	150	70
Classroom Work	150	100
Walking 4 mph	150	300
Cycling 5-10 mph	150	250-400
Farm Chores	150	230
Carpentry	150	230
Housepainting	150	200
Heavy Work	150	300-700
Domestic — from bedmaking to scrubbing	120	150-240
		CALORIES* per minute
Baseball	150	4.7
Basketball	160	8.0
Football	160	8.6
Pingpong	160	4.9
Tennis	150	7.0
Skiing	150	18.6
Sprinting	150	23.3

Calorie used is heat needed to raise the temperature of one kilogram (2.2 pounds) of water from 15° to 16° C.

OTHER TREATMENT MEASURES

Additional measures are recommended if dietary treatment fails to produce significant reduction in blood glucose levels, reflecting improved control and a reduction in the severity of D.M.

What is good control? It is a return of blood glucose values to normal, before and after eating (See p. 9).

What is satisfactory control? In some instances it may be satisfactory for blood glucose values to rise over 200 mg. per 100 ml. after eating, if there is absence of symptoms of D.M. and freedom from infections.

What is an unsatisfactory response? It is failure to reduce blood glucose values low enough to prevent excessive glucose loss in the urine, e.g. 10 to 20 grams in 24 hours. The loss of glucose stimulates the loss of water, salt and vitamins, causing disorders of nutrition and symptoms of diabetes. Under these circumstances it may be necessary to start: (a) insulin — turn to chapter 7; or (b) oral therapy — turn to chapter 6.

TREATMENT PROBLEMS

When dietary measures fail, it might be concluded that:

1. Diet instructions are not being carefully followed.

2. The overweight patient is not achieving weight reduction.

3. Other factors may be present, leading to resistance to insulin action. Many mild adult diabetics secrete quite adequate amounts of insulin. For this reason, it is difficult to accept the fact that the use of oral therapy or insulin will contribute to the care of this group of diabetic patients. However, in the presence of certain complications, your physician may wish to prescribe oral therapy (e.g. Orinase, Tolinase, Dymelor, Diabinese or DBI). At other times insulin may be indicated, particularly if a serious infection is present.

In 1971, the Federal Drug Administration (FDA) issued a warning suggesting that it may be dangerous to use the above-mentioned medications in the routine management of adult onset diabetes. This warning was issued following an eight-year study of orinase in the treatment of adult onset diabetes. This study was carried out in twelve university centers in this country. The warning was supported by the Council on Drugs of the American Medical Association and the American Diabetes Association. It produced evidence that after five or more years of use, Orinase treatment was associated with a higher incidence of deaths from heart disease (12.7 percent) than was diet treatment with a placebo (4.9 percent) or diet treatment with insulin (about 6 percent). Later the F.D.A. issued a similar warning about phenformin (DBI). The British and Canadian Diabetes Associations did not support this action of the F.D.A. In this country, the position of the F.D.A. was opposed by the Committee for the Care of the Diabetic. In February, 1975, the Biometrics Society, after a careful review of the data of the University Group Diabetes Program, reported their support of the conclusions developed by the U.G.D.P.

EVALUATING THE RESULTS OF TREATMENT

Treatment results can be measured in a number of specific ways:

1. Regular physician supervision with blood glucose checks.

2. Testing for glucose in the urine (See p. 108). It is suggested that urine passed 1-1/2 hours after one meal per day should be tested by those adult diabetic persons treated by diet alone or by diet and oral therapy. This will reveal any excessive rise in the blood glucose levels after eating. Testing of urine passed before the meal is less informative — most adult onset diabetics not requiring insulin have before-meal glucose values below that which leads to loss of glucose in the urine. As will be noted later, the insulin dependent diabetic is advised to test the second voided urine specimen before meals.

3. Regular checks of the effects of dietary management on weight control.

SUCCESS OF THE PROGRAM IS DEMONSTRATED BY:

1. Return to normal weight. Ideal weight may be determined by a formula suggested by Dr. Geo. Bray of Los Angeles:
   1) Ladies — Base weight of 100 pounds plus 5 pounds for each inch over 60 inches
   2) Men — Base weight of 106 pounds plus 6 pounds for each inch over 60 inches.

2. Return of blood glucose values to a satisfactory or normal range.

3. Evidence of confidence and accomplishment.

4. Freedom from complications that compromise good health, cause disability and work loss, and interfere with longevity.

DIETARY AND OTHER MODIFICATIONS FOR TREATMENT OF CO-EXISTENT ILLNESSES

1. The diabetic diet can be modified to allow treatment of:
   a. Heart disease with   1) low salt diet
   2) low fat diet
   b. Ulcer disease with milk and other modifications.
   c. Colitis with a bland diet for diarrhea. The recommended diet for those with symptoms of irritable colon is one that has a high fiber content eg., bran cereals, whole wheat bread.

2. Vitamins are often prescribed during periods of restricted food intake. They do not help to lose weight.

3. Most medications do not affect blood glucose values in this form of

D.M., but certain ones that might should be used only on prescription by a physician. These are:

Oral contraceptives
Thiazide diuretics
Nose drops and capsules for asthma containing EPINEPHRINE
Cortisone-containing medicines

4. There is little reason for concern about the use of the following medications when diabetes is managed **without** the use of oral anti-diabetic tablets:

Aspirin
Mild sedatives
Most tranquilizers
Arthritis medicines other than
    cortisone
Digitalis

Quinidine
Anticoagulants
Sugar-free cough medicines
Vitamins
Medications for diarrhea
Antacids

STEPS TO FOLLOW WHEN ACUTE ILLNESS AGGRAVATES ADULT ONSET D.M.

In the introduction it was recorded that certain conditions may precipitate signs or symptoms of diabetes. These same disorders can lead to an increase in severity of this form of diabetes. Once aware of this, what can be done?

1. Test urine for glucose regularly — even three to four times daily during an acute illness accompanied by fever.

2. If increasing amounts of glucose appear in the urine, consult with physician.

3. If loss of appetite occurs, use a liquid diet as instructed on page 116.

4. If nauseated, try 1/2 glass of 7-Up, Jello, broth or soup, or apple juice hourly (See p. 115).

5. Contact physician or his nurse clinician for additional suggestions. This is important for those on oral medication as well as for those requiring adjustment of insulin dose.

□ *ADDITIONAL MEASURES TO FOLLOW DURING ACUTE ILLNESS*

Regular test of urine for glucose.
If diabetes control becomes worse, consult physician.
For loss of appetite or nausea, change to liquid diet.
Consult physician for:
    stomach flu, fever, chest pain, foot lesion — in particular.

[1] Yalow, R. S. and Berson, S. A. (1960). Plasma Insulin Concentrations in Non-diabetic and Early Diabetic Subjects. *Diabetes* 9:254.

[2] Kipnis, D. M. (1968) Insulin Secretion in Diabetes Mellitus. *Annals of Int. Med.* 69:891.

[3] Siperstein, M. D. et al. (1968) Studies of Muscle Capillary Basement Membranes in Normal Subjects, Diabetic, and Prediabetic Patients. *Jour. Clin. Invest.* 47:1973.

[4] Williamson, J. R. in Kilo, C., et al. (1972) Muscle Capillary Basement Membrane Changes Related to Aging and to Diabetes Mellitus, *Diabetes* 21:881.

Chapter 2   JUVENILE OR INSULIN DEPENDENT DM

JUVENILE OR INSULIN DEPENDENT DIABETES MELLITUS

This chapter of the book is for the young diabetic and family members. It emphasizes the more sensitive nature of insulin dependent diabetes as reflected by: 1) sudden loss of controlled diabetes in relation to emotional upsets or acute infections; 2) significant drops in blood glucose leading to hypoglycemia (insulin reactions) when there is a delay in the meal hour or as a result of increased physical exertion.

WHAT DISTINGUISHES JUVENILE DIABETES MELLITUS?

Juvenile diabetes mellitus is different in many ways from adult onset diabetes (See pp. 17-23), yet both forms occur in the same families. Many reserve the term "juvenile diabetes" for those who develop diabetes before the age of 15 — others apply it not only to juveniles but also to adolescents and young adults who have complete insulin dependency. Juvenile diabetes frequently appears after an infection. Parents may note that the youngster is not regaining his health and, instead, has suddenly begun to have extreme thirst, frequency of urination, at times leading to bed-wetting, an increase in appetite accompanied by weight loss and fatigue, and failure of scratches and cuts to heal. If treatment is delayed, drowsiness and even coma may follow. It is usually preferable at this stage to admit the child to the hospital for treatment and for the parents to receive instruction in home management of diabetes.

☐ *SYMPTOMS OF JUVENILE DIABETES*

Thirst
Frequency of urination
Hunger
Weight loss
Fatigue
Delayed healing of lacerations, cuts
Eventually: Drowsiness, Coma

The symptoms of uncontrolled D.M. in the young diabetic are due to insulin deficiency, resulting in an excessive accumulation of glucose in the blood (See Fig. 2, p. 11). This, in turn, stimulates the kidneys to form large quantities of urine, resulting in frequency of passing urine and the loss of large amounts of glucose. The body becomes water-depleted, energy fades and body weight falls. Turn to page 10 for a more complete explanation.

OBJECTIVES OF TREATMENT

1. Relief of signs and symptoms of D.M.

2. Help the young diabetic understand and have control of the disease for the following reasons:

    a. A normal sense of well-being and security from health concerns.

    b. Normal growth and development.

    c. The capacity to resist certain infections.

    d. Prevention of complications, e.g.

        — Most important KETOACIDOSIS (See pp. 124-125).

        — Hypoglycemia (See p. 100).

        — Atherosclerosis — controlled diabetes helps to prevent high blood fat levels which may contribute to thickening of the walls of the arteries, i.e., atherosclerosis (See p. 127).

        — Neuritis (See p. 126).

        — Visual changes (See pp. 128-131).

TREATMENT OF JUVENILE DIABETES

Treatment means doing those things which help the young diabetic to once again feel well. An important part of the treatment is that which assists the youngster to accept the diagnosis and then to understand the nature of his illness. The job of the physician, then, is similar to that of the football or basketball coach who posts meetings and holds practices to inform, train, and motivate his team.* The winning coach develops not only alert and well-conditioned players but possibly the best disciplined team. These same criteria can be applied to help the young person manage diabetes. The best athletes stand out as they act quickly and instinctively. In other words, because of their training and experience they don't have to hesitate to think about every movement. Young people with D.M. must manage diabetes in a similar way. They should be so trained and encouraged that they will perform many of the treatment steps instinctively or routinely, thereby facilitating everyday living.

□ *CONTROL OF JUVENILE DIABETES IS SENSITIVE TO:*

    Variations in

Diet	Stress — Emotional
Exercise	Illness

*We recommend reading John Wooden — They Call Me Coach, Word Books, Waco, Texas. In it he describes his philosophy and definition of success. John Wooden's PYRAMID OF SUCCESS, is developed by use of building blocks containing key words, to build first a foundation, then additional tiers until the apex is formed: i.e., success. In the heart of the pyramid is the word condition.

□ *CONTROL OF JUVENILE DIABETES IS PROMOTED BY:*
   Regular eating habits
   Regular use of exercise
   Change in insulin dose in response to:
   — Hypoglycemic reactions
   — Poor diabetic control when due to
      emotional stress or acute illness

METHODS OF JUVENILE D.M. CONTROL

DIET

There are some differences among physicians about the degree and nature of diet in the management of juvenile diabetes. Of less controversy — any diet must be nutritious, i.e. supply vitamins, minerals, adequate protein for growth and calories for energy requirements and weight maintenance. Controversy centers on what degree of carbohydrate restriction is necessary in the diet. Unlimited intake leads to persistent elevation of glucose levels in the blood and heavy loss of glucose in the urine. Restriction of carbohydrates to a level where they contribute much less than 50 percent of the caloric intake is less palatable and undesirable.

The diet prescription must supply enough food for satisfaction and for energy needs. In addition to three meals, mid-day and bedtime snacks are beneficial. The snacks can help to prevent low blood glucose levels.

The diet can be constructed to conform to the individual and family eating patterns. Initially the diet should be either a weighed or household measure diet. After some experience with measuring it may be possible to become quite adept at estimating the diet.

Dietary details and instructions for use of the weighed calculated or exchange diets are presented in Part 2.

INSULIN

Prior to the last half century there were few great medical discoveries. Jenner developed the smallpox vaccination in the 1500's and Pasteur contributed to the science of bacteriology in the 1800's. Yet nothing prior to 1921 affected the lives of ill people as dramatically as did the discovery of insulin by Drs. Frederick Banting and Charles Best. For their research at the University of Toronto, Canada, they were awarded the Nobel Prize, a prize they shared with Drs. J. J. McLeod and J. B.

Collip. It is interesting that the first human to be kept alive by insulin injection was a 14-year-old boy. Leonard Thompson lay in deep coma on January 11, 1922, the day he first received insulin at the Toronto General Hospital. As a result of continuing insulin injections he regained consciousness and improved health.

Good nutrition and health are dependent upon the administration of insulin by injection in amounts that prevent excessive blood glucose levels, by promoting glucose uptake by tissue cells. It is not a cure for diabetes. Insulin must be injected one or more times a day. No other medicine or substance can be used in its place. It is not habit-forming, and the body rarely becomes resistant to its action. The directions for the use of insulin and other pertinent information can be found on pp. 84-100.

EXERCISE

Generally young diabetics can do whatever other young non-diabetics can do. This depends, however, on matching the insulin dose with physical activity and food intake. Physical activity and meal and snack times should be at regularly spaced intervals. During exercise the body uses glucose to supply energy. As the juvenile diabetic has limited stores of body sugar for energy, exercise may produce a fall in blood glucose level. This may be prevented by extra feedings before exercise. During strenuous exercise frequent use of a sweet liquid might be more advantageous. Such a routine may not be necessary during mild or moderate exercise if there has been difficulty maintaining control. In this case exercise may help establish control.

Regularity of exercise is difficult to maintain. Good weather invites much greater activity than poor weather. It follows that one may need more insulin to prevent loss of control during periods of less activity. On the other hand, one must accommodate for greater activity by using less insulin or more food. This will prevent the blood glucose from becoming too low, i.e. from becoming HYPOGLYCEMIC or having an insulin reaction (p. 100). It is important to know not only how to prevent hypoglycemia but recognize and treat, and quickly raise the blood glucose level.

DEVELOPMENT OF MENTAL ATTITUDE

A positive mental attitude is of assistance in overcoming some of the restrictions and other impositions resulting from having D.M. Acceptance of the diagnosis and learning how to treat diabetes are accomplishments. However, the greatest accomplishment is the firm decision to adopt and follow a recommended treatment program. The decision will later be recognized as worthwhile when it is found that the result is a good state of health, and the opportunity for a full and meaningful life. During this period of learning and maturing, children will be looking to their parents for support and guidance and to their physician for assistance and advice. The parents will be most helpful when they demonstrate a unified approach and show consistency in their advice.

Diabetic youngsters should be permitted the same courtesies, encouragements, attentions and disciplines as their non-diabetic peers. A sheltered or over-protected life or one that is characterized by neglect does not allow the child the opportunity to develop fully. Initially diabetic children, their parents and siblings need considerable help and guidance. This must be offered in a positive, thoughtful and constructive manner. Slowly, responsibilities for self-care should be transferred to the youngsters. As they gradually develop the ability and willingness to assume responsibility, the parents must relinquish their involvement. As the young diabetics achieve skill in giving injections, interpreting urine tests and estimating diets, the way is cleared for such activities as staying overnight with friends, travelling with the school team, and going camping. These further demonstrations of their accomplishments may well encourage these young people to be increasingly independent and faithful to their original goals.

STRESS

Acute stresses as exemplified by acute infection, acute emotional distress or pain trigger a number of reactions in the cells of our bodies. These responses help our bodies to withstand these stresses and recover from them. Among the responses are those which increase the amount of glucose in the blood and interfere with the action of insulin. Insulin-dependent diabetics may not tolerate this change as well as the non-diabetic. This will be demonstrated by the appearance of larger than usual amounts of sugar in the urine.

Many times acute stresses cannot be avoided. However, it is possible for many to manage some degree of accommodation to the lesser stresses, i.e. the concerns and conflicts that challenge us daily. If the young person tends to overreact to these common stresses, there will be more difficulty with the control of diabetes than if the diet was being neglected. Learning to cope with these experiences is called maturing.

Often the young diabetic discovers maturing is accompanied by more manageable diabetes. The management of diabetes during acute infections is covered on p. 115.

☐ *BLOOD GLUCOSE LEVEL INFLUENCED BY:*

Food Intake
    Quantity
    Irregularity of meals
Insulin
Exercise
Stress
   Emotional
   Illnesses accompanied by fever
   Injury leading to pain

THE RESULTS OF TREATMENT ARE MEASURED BY:

1. Return of a normal sense of well-being and the feeling of confidence that improves one's performance.

2. Maintenance of normal weight with adequate growth and development.

3. Freedom from those complications of poorly controlled diabetes which can interfere with one's state of health and performance.

Remission of severe diabetes to a milder state commonly occurs when treatment in the recently diagnosed diabetic reduces the blood glucose level. The remission, characterized by a significant decrease in insulin dose and diabetes which is easier to regulate, may last for weeks or months.

RESULTS ARE DEPENDENT ON:

1. Establishing a daily routine that reflects the recommendations of the treating physician. This includes:
    a. Regularity of meal hours, exercise and time of insulin injections.
    b. Keeping a record of daily urine tests for glucose (and ketones when indicated).
    c. Regular visits to the doctor for an interview, check of urine test records and body weight. When appropriate, a blood test for glucose and a measure of the glucose in a 24 hour urine specimen. Other parameters may also be reviewed.
    d. Checks of body weight at regular intervals.
    e. Contacting the physician early in the course of things if there is:
       1) A return of signs or symptoms of diabetes.

2) An acute infection.

3) Ketones in the urine with large amounts of glucose.

4) Hypoglycemia, if distressing or coming with some frequency.

SUMMER CAMPS FOR DIABETIC CHILDREN

It is not unusual today for diabetic children to attend non-diabetic summer camps or even to participate in wilderness survival programs. However, in 1925 it was unusual for a diabetic child to have any organized activity away from home. That year Dr. Leonard Wendt, recognizing a special need, operated a special camp for diabetic children. This was at a time when insulin had only been in use about three years, when ketoacidosis continually threatened and antibiotics were undreamed of. Although Dr. Wendt conducted the first camp for diabetic children, it was Dr. and Mrs. Henry John of Cleveland, Ohio, who established the first permanent camp for diabetic children in 1929. Since then the number of camps has increased and now every region of this country and Canada has a conveniently located camp. In many instances the camps are owned and operated by local diabetes associations. In other cases the diabetic camp program is operated in conjunction with that of other organizations.

There are many approaches to running summer camp programs. The late Dr. Lester Palmer of Seattle felt diabetic children benefited by camping with non-diabetic children. The Joslin Foundation has considered it appropriate to operate separate camps for boys and girls.

The Diabetic Children's Camp Foundation of Portland started its program in 1951. For the first three years established campsites were rented. Then in 1955 the Camp Foundation acquired property at Glenwood, Oregon, and established a permanent camp. Gales Creek Children's Camp admits both boys and girls by age groups. At Gales Creek Camp, as at other camps in the country, no child is refused admission because of inability to pay any portion of the camp fee.

The objectives of the program are:

1. To encourage the children by example, education and association to learn and use those skills that will assist them in better medical control of their diabetes.

2. To provide medical facilities sufficient to help re-establish control in some children who might otherwise have to be hospitalized after the school year.

3. To present recreational programs which are challenging and stimulating as well as enjoyable. As a result of their participation in many of these activities, diabetic children develop a greater appreciation of their physical potential.

4. To provide instruction in the camp medical center in urine testing, insulin injection technique, and in group discussions to assist in better understanding of diabetes and some of the problems of living with diabetes. An important phase of the discussions is the opportunity the campers have to discuss their concerns with each other.

5. To give the youngsters some time away from home in an environment which encourages them to become more self-reliant and more independent. Of course, this is also a time for the parents and guardians to relax and become refreshed. After some experience at diabetic summer camp it will be quite natural for many children to branch out into other summer activities and for their parents to feel supportive of these moves.

A list of the diabetic summer camps operational in the United States and their location is available from The American Diabetes Association, Inc., 1 West 48th Street, New York, N.Y. 10020.

Information about camps in Canada may be obtained from: The Canadian Diabetic Association, 1491 Yonge Street, Toronto, Ontario, 10, Canada.

Part 2

DIETARY MANAGEMENT

DIETARY MANAGEMENT OF DM
— General Comments —

DIETS AND D.M.

It has been emphasized that control of diabetes is desirable and that there should be awareness of the factors that lead to uncontrolled diabetes. The insulin-dependent diabetic often reveals considerable sensitivity to physical exercise, emotional distress and acute infection. The influence of these factors is better tolerated in those persons who have adhered to a diet plan and can adjust their diet in relation to the demands of increased physical activity or necessary restrictions during acute illness. Those who do not require insulin may develop milder diabetes by dietary management and weight control. From these observations it is evident that the diabetic diet is the key to the successful management of diabetes.

CHARACTERISTICS OF DIABETIC DIETS

1. Sweets are excluded and some restriction of carbohydrate foods is desirable. A measured amount of protein is recommended, particularly for the young diabetic, to insure adequate growth and development. Supplementary vitamins are not usually required when the dietary recommendations are followed and the diabetes is adequately controlled. Vitamins are advised for those on a low calorie diet or those with uncontrolled diabetes.

2. The diet prescription of carbohydrate, protein and fat (C-P-F) is designed to be adequate in calorie content and to offer foods supplying adequate nutrients, such as minerals and vitamins. If a low calorie diet is prescribed it is followed until sufficient weight control has taken place.

3. The diet can be measured as:
   A. Calculated weighed or weighed exchange diet.
   B. American Diabetes Association (A.D.A.) diet.
The diet should be constant in amount from day to day. If insulin is required, regularity of meal hours is also important.

4. As most foods can be eaten, efforts should be made to make the diet attractive and palatable. In most cases it can be adjusted to meet individual tastes and food habits.

5. The diet should include directions for:

A. Switching to a liquid diet during acute feverish illnesses and gastroenteritis.
B. Use of additional or larger snacks during and after such periods of excessive activity as gardening, mountain climbing, golfing, jogging, and dancing.
C. Use of extra carbohydrates intermittently during such continuous and strenuous activities as basketball, hockey, football, and aggressive tennis.

Many people in this country have erratic eating habits based upon convenience rather than good nutrition. It may be difficult for these persons to make the necessary adjustments to regular hours for eating and to include many of the foods that are conducive to good health and nutrition.

GUIDELINES FOR FOLLOWING A DIABETIC DIET

1. Most foods should be measured after they are cooked.

2. All vegetables should be cooked without fat, unless it is permitted in the diet. Use fresh, frozen or canned vegetables.

3. Fruits should be fresh, unsweetened frozen or canned fruits or juices.

4. Cook meats by roasting, broiling in pan or broiler, stewing, or simmering. Trim off visible fat.

5. Artificial sweeteners e.g. saccharin are used with the advice of the physician.

6. There are a number of free foods that do not have to be worked into the diet.

DIET PRESCRIPTION

The diet prescription is determined by the physician to supply the necessary caloric requirement (carbohydrate, protein and fat) of the patient. Within a fairly wide range, this also can be adjusted by the physician to meet individual tastes and food habits.

For the young patient with diabetes the diet prescription must permit adequate growth and development. For the older patient with diabetes the diet prescription is necessary for maintaining or achieving normal weight. The diet prescription is also necessary in helping a patient eat the same quantity of food each day to promote better control of diabetes.

CALORIES

A calorie is a unit of heat which corresponds to an equivalent amount of energy. Foods furnish calories in the following amounts:

1 gram Carbohydrate supplies .... 4 calories of energy
1 gram Protein supplies .... 4 calories of energy
1 gram Fat supplies .... 9 calories of energy
1 gram Alcohol supplies .... 7 calories of energy

Food taken in larger amounts than necessary to meet the body's energy requirement is eventually converted to fat with a resulting increase in body weight. When insufficient food is eaten to meet the energy needs, the body can then reconvert this stored fat to energy.

A diet should have sufficient calories to supply energy needs and maintain normal weight.

BALANCED DIET

A daily menu containing the following will roughly meet the above requirements, and, in addition, supply the vitamins and minerals necessary for proper utilization of the diet.

Milk .... 1 to 2 pints daily
Egg, or a serving of cheese .... 1 daily
Fruit..................................... 1 to 2 servings daily
Meat .... 1 or more servings daily
Bread and Cereal .... 3 servings daily
Vegetable (including 1 serving of green or yellow
    leafy vegetable, raw) .... 2 or more servings daily

CARBOHYDRATE

In food, carbohydrate exists either in sugar or starch, all of which is broken down by the body to glucose, a simple sugar. The primary function of carbohydrate is to serve as a source of body energy. Any excess (over what the body needs for energy) is converted to fat. They are found in fruits, vegetables, cereal, bread, and many dairy products.

PROTEIN

Protein is the basic constituent of body tissue, and varying amounts are necessary in the diet for replacement of "wear and tear" of body tissues. Any excess, over the amount needed for replacement of body tissues, is readily converted to sugar by the body and eventually to fat. Proteins are found in meat, eggs, fish, milk products, cereal, bread, and nuts, with small amounts in vegetables.

FAT

Fat also serves as a source of energy, somewhat more slowly available than carbohydrate, and any excess is stored as body fat. Fats are found chiefly in diary products, oils, margarine, eggs, meat, and nuts. A certain minimum amount of so-called "essential fats" is necessary in a well balanced diet, but the unusually high fat content of food consumed in prosperous "civilized" countries is the chief cause of obesity and may be a factor in the early development of hardening of the arteries.

CALCULATED DIETS

Diet calculation allows a patient greater freedom within the diet prescription. With a knowledge of food values and an understanding of the simple arithmetic necessary, the patient may construct a diet around his individual food preferences.

By calculating his own diet, the patient has greater freedom to vary his menus — limited only by how much time the patient is willing to spend calculating various combinations. Since all diabetic diets are really based on the calculated-weighed diet, it is our feeling that all patients benefit from this approach initially even though some other approach may be used in the day-to-day management of diabetes.

Furthermore, it is possible to use special recipes for casseroles, some desserts and various prepared foods which are usually excluded from diabetic diets.

EXCHANGE DIETS

Exchange diets consist of various exchange food lists, which are so constructed that one food can be substituted for another of the list by using the designated amount. The number of servings and the specific amount of each food either in gram weight or household measurement are recorded for each meal.

The exchange diet relieves the patient of the necessity for diet calculation but does restrict the patient's choice to a certain degree. Time and again, however, we have been impressed that patients understand their exchange diets much better after they have learned the principles of diet calculation. Although the weighed exchange diet is more accurate, the household measure exchange diet may be adequate, particularly in the relatively mild and stable diabetes where weight control is not a problem. Certainly a household exchange diet which is understood and followed consistently may well be more satisfactory than a calculated-weighed diet for the patient who has neither the time nor inclination to follow the regimen consistently.

METRIC SYSTEM

In many instances a weighed diet will be prescribed, therefore it is necessary to understand the following weights and measurements.

Gram: A gram is a unit of dry weight in the Metric System.

Table for measuring or weighing liquids of a density of water:

5 grams	=	1 tsp.
15 grams	=	3 tsp. or 1 tbsp.
30 grams	=	2 tbsp. or 1 ounce
113 grams	=	4 ounces or 1/2 cup
227 grams	=	8 ounces or 1 cup
454 grams	=	16 ounces or 2 cups or 1 pint

Table for measuring or weighing dry foods:

Flour:

			Sugar-Twin:		
2 grams	=	1 tsp.	1 gram	=	1 tbsp.
6 grams	=	3 tsp. or 1 tbsp.	8 grams	=	1/3 cup
45 grams	=	1/3 cup	13 grams	=	1/2 cup
70 grams	=	1/2 cup	25 grams	=	1 cup

Solid foods weigh quite differently from each other, therefore it is often necessary to weigh various ingredients of a recipe in order to have accurate food values. In general, one pound of solid food weighs approximately 453 grams.

EQUIPMENT SUGGESTIONS FOR USING A WEIGHED OR MEASURED DIET

The Hansen 500 gram food scales are recommended for a weighed diet. These scales are graduated in grams and have a movable indicator so that the pointer may be moved back to zero after each food is added, allowing more than one food to be weighed without removing the plate from the scales. Use a plastic, paper, or other lightweight plate for weighing foods. The usual china dinner plate is too heavy for use on these scales.

A weighed diet (either calculated or exchange) offers the obvious advantage of greater accuracy and consistency. The physician may feel that this is indicated for best control of diabetes in certain cases and it is most important where weight control is a real problem.

Using gram scales takes the guess work out of a diet. There is no such thing as an average slice of bread or a medium size potato. After sufficient training with the gram scales at home, it is easier to estimate servings when eating out.

The household measure diet requires the use of an 8 ounce measuring cup, a measuring teaspoon and tablespoon. All measures are level measures.

WASTE OF FOODS

With some foods, it is difficult to weigh the edible portion only and still serve an appealing product. For estimating the percentage of waste, use the following guidelines:

Apple core 10%
Apple skin and core 15%
Apricot pit 10%
Artichoke refuse 50%
Banana peel 30%
Cherry pit 10%
Chicken bones:
    Neck, drumstick, wing 50%
    Thigh 25%
    Breast 20%
Coconut shell 50%
Corn cob 50%
Egg shell 10%
Grape stem and seeds 10%
Grapefruit rind 50%
Nut shells 50%
Olive pit 50%
Orange peel 50%
Plum pit 10%
Prune pit 15%
Salmon steak bone 10%
Shrimp shell 30%
Watermelon rind 50%

FOODS TO AVOID

Sugar	Candy
Honey	Sweet pickles
Jams, Jellies, Preserves	Fried foods unless additional
Syrups	fat is allowed in diet

Fruit, canned or frozen with sugar
Gelatin made with sugar (except in Liquid Diet)
Regular carbonated beverages (except in Liquid Diet)
Deserts made with sugars (with the exception of ice cream and some low calorie cookies)

FREE FOODS (Allowed as desired)

Boullion	Horse Radish	Vinegar
Clear Broth	Mustard	D-Zerta Gelatin
Coffee	Spices	All artificial sweet-
Tea	Herbs	eners (except lo-
		calorie sugars)
		Vanilla and other
		flavorings

DIETETIC LOW CALORIE FOODS

Foods to be used in moderate amounts (20 free calories a day)
Artificially sweetened jams, jellies, and syrups
Carbonated beverages (where no sugar added)
Catsup
Sugarless gum
Low calorie (low fat) salad dressings, mayonnaise, and chocolate sauce.

Some brand names of products which are low-calorie are listed below. Be certain to read the label for the number of calories per serving. If there are less than 20 calories per serving, it may be used from the **20 free calories a day.**

Tillie Lewis — syrups, jams and jellies, catsup, chocolate sauce
S&W Nutradiet — jams and jellies, syrup
Harvey's — gum
Trident — gum
Care-Free — gum
Clark's Di-et — gum
Estee — gum, bubble gum, fruit drops
Amurol — fruit drops, mints
Cary's — syrup

Remember the word **dietetic** does not mean **diabetic.** Many dietetic food products are for use with low salt or low cholesterol diets. **Dietetic** foods which may be used in **diabetic** diet plans usually are not to be used freely, but must be figured into the diet.

The caloric values given on the label of standard food products is not very helpful. However, when using a small amount of a **dietetic** food product such as sugarless gum, jelly or carbonated beverage, the caloric value is a good guideline.

Example: S&W Strawberry Jam: 1 teaspoon = 4 calories.

DIETETIC SUGARLESS FOODS

These are foods to be used with caution. They are sweetened with Sorbitol and Mannitol; they are sugarless but are a starchy carbohydrate and are not necessarily low caloric. In most cases they do have to be figured into the diet, such as

Dietetic (sugar-free) ice cream
Dietetic (sugar-free) cookies
Dietetic (sugar-free) candy

For example, one small dietetic candy bar has approximately 116 calories from 7 grams carbohydrate, 4 grams protein, and 8 grams of fat.

INFORMATION ON LABELS

It is important to know how to use various food items in diet planning. Prepared products can often be used when the food values are known. In recent months legislation has required more complete labeling which allows more freedom in the use of these products. Then it becomes necessary to understand the values given in the label information.

It is also important to watch for key words like sucrose, lactose, dextrin or dextrose (which are types of sugars); sorbitol, mannitol (which are types of starches with a sweet taste); lo-calorie (which may have nothing to do with sugar, but may be low in fat, or may be lower in sugar, but not be sugar-free). The accompanying label information should be stated so that it is possible to know either the carbohydrate, protein and fat value in a stated size of serving, or the number of calories in a stated size of serving.

Below are some examples of label information and their interpretation:

CHICKEN OF THE SEA: Chunk Light Tuna (packed in vegetable oil)
Portion Size — Total Can Contents (6½ oz.-190 gms.)
Calories (including oil) 470
Carbohydrate 1 gm.
Protein 45 gms.
Fat (including oil) 32 gms.

Percentage of U.S. Recommended Daily Allowance: This information is important from a nutritional standpoint, but is not necessary for figuring the C-P-F value of the food.

If the whole can of tuna (including oil) was eaten, C-1, P-45, F-32 would be used. This is the same as 5 meat and 3 fat exchanges.

The drained weight of the tuna is: 160 gms. (30 gms. of oil and water was removed, which, in this instance was approximately 15 gms. of fat) or C-1, P-45, F-17. The value per 100 gms. is C-1, P-22, F-7; per 30 gm. serving: C-0, P-7, F-2. This is approximately equal to 1 meat exchange.

GREEN GIANT NIBLETS: Whole Kernel Golden Corn
Serving Size — 1 cup (6 oz., which is approximately 180 gms.)
Calories 150
Carbohydrate 35 gms.
Protein 3 gms.
Fat 2 gms.
This works out to be approximately C-20, P-2, F-0 per 100 gms. of corn. 1 bread exchange would weigh 75 gms.

FRANCO AMERICAN SPAGHETTI IN TOMATO SAUCE w/CHEESE
Serving Size: (7½ oz., or 213 gms.)
Calories 180

Carbohydrate	34 gms.		16	
Protein	5 gms.	=	3	per 100 gms., or
Fat	2 gms.		1	1 bread exchange

CAMPBELL'S OLD FASHIONED TOMATO RICE SOUP
Serving Size: 5 oz. (156 gm.) condensed

Calories:	130			
Carbohydrate	25		18	
Protein	2	=	1	per 100 gms., or
Fat	3		1	2 soup exchange

ARTIFICIAL SWEETENERS

In 1969 the marketing of cyclamate compounds and solutions for use as artificial sweeteners ceased by authority of the Federal Drug Administration. Since then efforts to fill the void have led to increased use of low calorie sugars and the older agents such as saccharin, sorbitol and mannitol.

Low-calorie sugars, though recommended for use by those with diabetes, cannot be freely consumed. They contain dextrose and lactose and thus have carbohydrate food value. Many of them have filler substances which decreases the carbohydrate value by weight. It is possible to use these sugars as a sweetener for beverages and cereal, but the preferable use is in baking. The end product will have a much better texture because sugar rather than a chemical sweetener was used. The low-calorie sugar adds to the carbohydrate value of the baked goods.

Sorbitol is a chemical compound of the sugar plus alcohol class. It is therefore a carbohydrate and has caloric value. It is used as a sweetening agent in dietetic candies, jellies, jams, some ice creams, and other specially prepared foods. Each gram of sorbitol generates four calories.

Saccharin is a non-caloric sweetener which can be added to foods that are not to be frozen or cooked. Either process causes deterioration of saccharin resulting in materials that lead to a bitter taste. Most liquid sweetening agents, e.g. Sucaryl, Jellsweet, Sweet 10, Superose, now contain saccharin. Saccharin is used in such sprinkler products as Adolph's sugar substitute and, of course, is still available in 1/4 and 1/2 grain tablets.

SWEETENERS

	Calories	Amount	Sugar Equivalent
POWDER — LACTOSE PREPARATIONS			
Necta Sweet	3	1 pkg.	2 tsp.
Sweetness & Light*	3½	1 tsp.	1 tsp.
Sweet'n Low	3	1 pkg.	2 tsp.
— SACCHARIN & LACTOSE			
Adolph's Sugar Substitute	2	2 shakes	1 tsp.
Superose	4	1 pkg.	2 tsp.
LIQUID — SACCHARIN			
Abbot Sucaryl	0	1/8 tsp.	1 tsp.
Adolph's Liquid Gold	0	1/8 tsp.	1 tsp.
Sweet 10	0	1/8 tsp.	1 tsp.
GRANULATED SUGAR REPLACEMENT			
Dextrin plus saccharin			
Sprinkle Sweet*	2	1 tsp.	1 tsp.
Sugar Twin*	2	1 tsp.	1 tsp.

*100 Gm = contains 93 grams carbohydrate.

Chapter 3 THE CALCULATED DIET

RULES FOR DIET CALCULATION

Diet Prescription:

The diet prescription gives the amount of carbohydrate, protein and fat allowed for one day. The amount of one meal is usually 1/3 of the daily allowance although, under certain circumstances, your physician may prescribe a different apportionment of the daily diet, e.g.,

Diet prescription C-150; P-90; F-30

Each Meal .... C- 50; P-30; F-10

Food Value Table:

These tables tell you the number of grams of carbohydrate, protein and fat in 100 grams of each food listed. For examples:

Bread C-53, P-9; F-2

This means that in 100 grams of bread there are:
53 grams of carbohydrate or 53% carbohydrate
9 grams of protein or 9% protein
2 grams of fat or 2% fat

You will notice that the total number of grams of carbohydrate, protein and fat (53 plus 9 plus 2) for 100 grams of bread adds up to only 64 grams. The difference (36 gms.) is made up by water and non-absorbable fibers with no food value.

Diet Calculation Involves Two Basic Determinations:

1. Figuring the amount of carbohydrate, protein and fat in a given portion of food, and

2. Determining the size serving of food necessary to supply a given amount of carbohydrate, protein or fat.

Since both of the calculations involve values for 1 gram of food, the first step is to determine the C.P. and F. for one gram of food.

Determination of amount of carbohydrate, protein and fat in one gram of food.

Since the food values express the amount of carbohydrate, protein and fat in 100 grams of food, to determine the amount in 1 gram, divide by 100.

Value for 100 gms of bread:
  C 53   P 9   F 2
Value for 1 gm. of bread:
  C 53/100   P 9/100   F 2/100

Using the decimal system, this is accomplished by moving the decimal point two places to the left.

Value for 100 gms. of bread:
  C 53   P 9   F 2
Value for 1 gm. of bread:
  C .53   P .09   F .02

To determine the amount of carbohydrate, protein and fat in a given serving of food.

1. Weigh the food

2. Multiply the weight of the serving by the amount of carbohydrate, protein, and fat in 1 gm. of food.

3. Round off to nearest whole number.

i.e., bread weight of serving 30 gms.
Amount of C .53, P .09 and F .02 in one gm. of bread.
Serving contains:
  30 X .53 = 15.9 gm. carbo.
  30 X .09 = 2.7 gm. protein
  30 X .02 =   .60 gm. fat
C16, P3, F1 in 30 gms. of bread

Determining the amount of a given food necessary to use up a given number of grams of carbohydrate, protein or fat.

1. Divide the number of grams of carbohydrate (or protein or fat) by the amount of carbohydrate (or protein or fat) in one gram of the food in question.

2. Round off to nearest whole number.

3. Multiply the weight of the serving arrived at by the amount of protein and fat in one gram of the carbohydrate food, or by the amount of fat in 1 gm. of protein food.

20 gms. of carbohydrate to be used up as bread.

1 gm. of bread contains .53 gms. of carbohydrate.
  .53 / 20.00

        37.7- grams of bread
  53 / 2000   to use up 20
       159   grams of carbo-
       410   hydrate.
       371
       390

38 X .09 = 3.42 gm. protein
38 X .02 = .76 gm. fat

SUMMARY OF RULES FOR DIET CALCULATION.

1. Divide the total C.P.F. by 3 to obtain the number of grams of each allowed for each meal. For example:

```
 C   P   F
180  90  60  ................... Total allowance for the day
 60  30  20  ................... Allowance for each meal
```

2. List the foods desired for each meal in the following groups:
   A. Carbohydrate foods first. Some foods containing carbohydrate will also contain protein and fat, but must be listed under carbohydrate foods.
   B. Protein foods second. The value for the protein contained in the carbohydrate foods will be subtracted from the protein allowance. The amount of protein left will be available for the protein foods.
   C. Fat foods third. In this list will be foods containing fat only, such as butter. The amount of fat available for this group will be determined by the fat left over after subtracting the fat in the carbohydrate and protein foods from the allowance for the meal.

3. To find the food value of a serving of food:
   A. Weigh the desired portion on the scale to get the weight in grams.
   B. Multiply the weight in grams by the value for 1 gram of food. For example:
   70 grams of potato:
       Value for 100 grams is 18-3-0
       Value for 1 gram is .18-.03-0

C	P
70	70
.18	.03
5.60	2.1
7.0	
12.60	

Round off to nearest whole number, so value for 70 grams of potato is:

      C-13   P-2   F-0

4. Subtract the C.P. and F. of each serving from the allowance for the meal in the order calculated. (See sample diet calculation.)

5. When you reach the last food in the carbohydrate list, you determine the amount of this food allowed by dividing the grams of carbohydrate allowance left by the carbohydrate value for 1 gram of the food. For example:

```
Bread —                                              C   P   F
Value for 100 grams ............................ 53   9   2
Value for 1 gram ................................ .53
```
15 grams of carbohydrate allowance left for bread.
.53/ 15 equals 28 grams of bread to use up carbohydrate allowance.

SAMPLE DIET

(Total carbohydrate 180; protein 90; fat 60)

Food	Value/100 Gms. C	P	F	Weight Serving	C (60)	P (30)	F (20)
Lettuce (3%)	Not calculated			30			
Potato	18	3	0	100	18	3	0
					42	27	20
Peas	9	3	0	80	7	2	0
					35	25	20
Milk	5	3	4	100	5	3	4
					30	22	16
Grapes	15	1	0	100	15	1	0
					15	21	16
Bread	53	9	2	28	15	3	1
					0	18	15
Beef Roast	0	30	6	60		18	4
						0	11
Olive oil dressing	0	0	100	5			5
							6
Butter	0	0	80	7			6
							0

CONVERSION TABLE: is available to simplify arriving at weights of food or amounts in grams carbohydrate, protein or fat in food during diet calculation.

FOOD VALUES FOR CALCULATED DIETS

CARBOHYDRATE FOODS

1. VEGETABLES

Food values for 100 grams of vegetables. Values are for canned, fresh, frozen, or cooked vegetables.

Average serving: Varies from 70 to 100 grams.

For purposes of diet calculation protein values of 3 or less need not be considered.

3% Vegetables C-3, P-1, F-0
           (C-.03; P-.01; F-.0 for 1 gram)
   (Up to 150 gm. per meal need not be calculated in diet.)

Asparagus	Egg plant	Sauerkraut
Bamboo shoots	Greens	String beans
Broccoli	Lettuce	Squash, summer
Cabbage	Mushrooms	Tomatoes
Cauliflower	Parsley	Tomato juice
Celery	Pepper, green	V-8 Vegetable juice
Chives	Pimentoes	Watercress
Cucumber	Radish	Zucchini
Dill pickles	Romaine	

6% Vegetables C-6, P-3, F-0
           (C-.06; P-.03; F-.0 for 1 gram)

Carrots (cooked, canned, or frozen)	Pumpkin
	Turnips
Okra	Brussel sprouts
Onions (cooked, canned)	Rutabagas

9% Vegetables C-9, P-3, F-0
           (C-.09; P-.03; F-.0 for 1 gram)

*Artichokes (French or Jerusalem — freshly harvested)	Leeks
	Okra, frozen
Bean sprouts	Onions, raw
Beets	Peas, fresh or frozen
Carrots, raw	Squash, winter (boiled or frozen)
Italian beans	Tomato puree (sauce)

*Artichokes — with storage, insulin conversion to available carbohydrate increases carbohydrate value to as much as 47 grams. (Jerusalem)

12% Vegetables C-12, P-3, F-0
        (C-.12; P-.03; F-.0 for 1 gram)

Hominy	Peas, canned
Mixed frozen vegetables	Squash, winter (baked)
Parsnips	

18% Vegetables C-18, P-3, F-0
        (C-.18; P-.03; F-.0 for 1 gram)

Artichokes, Jerusalem	Potatoes (mashed, baked, boiled)
Corn (canned, frozen, fresh)	Water chestnuts
Lima beans (canned)	Succotash
	Tomato paste

High Carbohydrate Vegetables	C	P	F
Beans			
Baked beans	20	6	0
Pork and beans	20	6	5
Kidney beans, canned	16	6	0
Kidney beans, dried and cooked	20	8	0
Lima beans, dried and cooked	24	8	0
Lima beans, frozen	20	7	0
Garbanzas, dried and cooked	20	8	2
Corn, cream style	20	2	0
Potatoes			
French fried potatoes	36	4	13
French fried potatoes, frozen	33	4	8
Potato chips	49	5	40
Sweet potatoes, boiled	26	2	0
Sweet potatoes, baked	32	2	0
Split peas, cooked	20	8	0
Soybeans			
Soybean curd (tofu)	2	8	4
Soybeans			
Immature seeds, cooked, boiled, drained	10	10	5
Mature seeds, raw	34	34	18
Mature seeds, cooked	11	11	6
Sprouted seeds, cooked, boiled, drained	4	5	1

2. FRUITS

Food values for 100 grams of fruit.
Use fresh or water-packed (W.P.) with or without artificial sweetening.
Do not use commercially frozen fruit unless label says no sugar added.

Average serving of fruit is 100 grams.

Average serving of fruit juice is 120 grams or 1/2 cup.

For purposes of diet calculation protein value of fruit may be ignored and given zero value.

There are some fruits which are lower than 6% carbohydrate, but may vary depending upon the preparation method. Be sure to check the label of commercially prepared products.

4% Fruits
    Low calorie cranapple juice
    Rhubarb, fresh

5% Fruits
    Low calorie cranberry juice (has a small amount of sugar in it with artificial sweetener)

6% Fruits C-6, P-1, F-0
        (C-.06; P-.01; F-.0 for 1 gram)

Blackberries, W.P.	Loganberries, W.P.	Strawberries
Cantaboupe	Mandarin oranges, W.P.	Watermelon
Grapefruit, W.P.	Peaches, W.P.	
Honeydew melon	Raspberries, W.P.	

9% Fruits C-9, P-1, F-0
        (C-.09; P-.01; F-.0 for 1 gram)

Applesauce	Grapefruit	Papayas
Apricots, W.P.	Grapefruit, juice pak	Peaches
Blackberries	Greengage plums, W.P.	Pears, W.P.
Boysenberries	Guavas	Pineapple. W.P.
Cranberries	Lemons	Raspberries
Fruit cocktail, W.P.	Lemon juice	
Gooseberries	Lime	
Grapefruit juice	Lime juice	

12% Fruits C-12, P-1, F-0
        (C-.12; P-.01; F-.0 for 1 gram)

Apple juice	Peach nectar
Apricots	Pear nectar
Cherries, W.P.	Pineapple
Cider, unsweetened	Pineapple juice
Figs, W.P.	Plums
Loganberries	Plums, W.P.
Oranges	Tangerines
Orange juice	
Peaches, juice pak	

15% Fruits C-15, P-1, F-0
        (C-.15; P-.01; F-.0 for 1 gram)

Apples	Grapes	Pomegranates
Apricot nectat	Huckleberries	Pears
Blueberries	Mangos	Pineapple, juice pak

18% Fruits C-18, P-1, F-0
        (C-.18; P-.01; F-.0 for 1 gram)

Cherries, sweet	Nectarines
Figs	Prune juice
Grape juice	Plums, purple (prunes)

Dried Fruits (Uncooked)	C	P	F
Apples	69	1	2
Apricots	63	5	1
Currants	74	2	2
Dates	71	2	1
Figs	64	4	1
Prunes	66	2	1
Raisins	77	3	0

Other Fruits	C	P	F
Avocado	5	2	16
Chinese Gooseberries	30	1	0
Prunes (cooked with no sugar)	32	2	0
Banana	22	1	0
Dried Apricots (cooked with no sugar)	21	2	0

3. BREAKFAST CEREALS

Carbohydrate foods with weights and food values for servings commonly used. The household measure is useful, but for times when greater accuracy is needed, use gram scales.

Food values for 100 grams of cereal and food values and weights for average servings.

Household Measurement	Gram Weight	C	P	F
All Bran	100	60	13	3
1/2 cup	30	18	4	1
Bran Flakes	100	71	10	2
1/2 cup	30	22	4	1
Cheerios	100	71	13	7
1 cup	25	17	4	1

(3 Cont.)

Household Measurement	Gram Weight	C	P	F
Corn Chex	100	86	7	2
Corn Flakes	100	85	8	0
1 cup	25	21	2	0
Cornmeal (cooked)	100	11	1	0
1/2 cup	135	15	1	0
Cream of Wheat (cooked)	100	9	1	0
1/2 cup	135	12	1	0
Grape Nuts	100	86	10	1
1/2 cup	30	25	3	0
Grape Nut Flakes	100	82	10	1
3/4 cup	30	23	4	0
Kix	100	84	9	2
Krumbles	100	82	9	1
1/2 cup	30	25	3	0
Oatmeal (cooked)	100	10	2	1
1/2 cup	150	15	3	2
Oatmeal (dry)	100	67	14	7
1 cup (dry)	85	64	9	1
Puffed Rice	100	77	15	2
1 cup	13	11	1	0
Puffed Wheat	100	76	17	2
1 cup	12	9	2	0
Raisin Bran (2/3 cup)	30	22	2	1
Rice Chex	100	88	6	0
1 cup	30	25	2	0
Rice Krispies	100	82	6	0
1 cup	25	22	2	0
Shredded Wheat	100	79	10	2
1 cup (spoon size)	40	32	4	1
1 biscuit	22	17	2	0
Special K	100	78	20	0
1 cup	20	14	4	0
Team	100	86	6	2
1 cup	30	24	2	1
Wheaties	100	79	10	2
1 cup	30	23	3	1

4 CEREAL PRODUCTS AND FLOURS

Household Measurement	Gram Weight	C	P	F
Barley, pearled (dry)	100	78	8	1
2 tbsp.	28	22	2	0
Bisquick	100	69	8	13
1 cup	120	78	11	15
Chow Mein Noodles	100	58	13	24
Cornmeal (dry)	100	78	8	1
1 cup	145	113	13	1
Cornstarch	100	88	0	0
1 tbsp.	8	7	0	0
Flour, white	100	75	11	1
1 cup	110	83	12	1
1 tbsp.	8	6	1	0
Hominy (dry)	100	78	8	1
1 cup	160	125	14	1
Macaroni (cooked)	100	23	3	0
1/2 cup	70	16	2	0
Noodles (cooked)	100	23	4	2
1/2 cup	80	18	3	2
Pancakes (cooked)	100	32	7	7
1 average 4" dia.	45	14	3	3
Pancake Mix (dry), Betty Crocker ...	100	80	8	0
1 cup	125	91	11	2
Pancake Mix (dry), Aunt Jemima	100	72	9	0
1 cup	111	80	11	1
Rice (cooked)	100	23	2	0
1/2 cup	84	19	2	0
Spaghetti (cooked)	100	23	3	0
1/2 cup	73	17	3	0
Tortilla	100	45	5	2
1 cake	10	5	1	0
Tapioca, dry	100	83	1	0
1 tbsp.	10	9	0	0
Waffles (frozen) round	100	42	7	6
1 waffle	48	19	3	4
Wheat Germ	100	44	27	11
1 tbsp.	100	4	2	1

5. BREAD, CRACKERS & SNACK LIST

Household Measurement	Gram Weight	C	P	F
Bread (white, rye, whole wheat, raisin, etc.)	100	53	9	2
1 average slice	30	16	3	1
1 thin slice	22	12	2	0
1 hard roll	35	19	3	1
1 soft roll	30	16	3	1
1 hamburger or frankfurter roll	50	27	5	1
Bread (low calorie)				
Hollywood Diet, 1 slice	18	9	2	0
Langendorf Vita-High Protein, 1 slice	19	8	2	1
Pepperidge Farm, 1 slice	24	12	2	1
Profile, 1 slice	23	10	2	1
Angelfood Cake, baked (plain)	100	60	7	0
Arrow Root Biscuits	100	72	6	10
2 biscuits	10	7	1	1
Barnum's Animal Crackers	100	78	5	3
6 crackers	12	10	1	1
Cheez-it Crackers	100	56	12	26
10 crackers	11	6	1	3
Cornbread, average package mix or recipe	100	33	6	8
Corn Chips	100	51	6	38
Donuts, cake type, plain	100	51	5	19
1 donut	40	20	2	8
Ginger Snaps	100	81	5	10
3 small	9	7	0	1
Graham Crackers, Sugar Honey	100	77	7	11
2 crackers	14	11	1	2
Ice Cream Cones	100	77	10	2
1 average cone	5	4	1	0
Lorna Doone Shortbread Cookies ...	100	66	6	27
2 cookies	16	10	1	4
Melba Toast	100	73	13	6
2 pieces	8	6	1	0
Popcorn, popped	100	75	13	5
1 cup	14	11	2	1

(5 Cont.) Household Measurement	Gram Weight	C	P	F
Pretzels	100	78	9	4
5 pretzels	16	12	1	1
Approx. 20 sticks	10	8	1	0
Ritz Crackers	100	60	6	30
4 crackers	12	7	1	4
Ry-Krisp	100	74	13	1
2 crackers	13	10	2	0
Saltines	100	72	9	12
2 crackers	6	4	1	1
5 crackers	15	11	1	2
Sponge cake, baked (plain)	100	54	8	6
Sunflower Seed Kernels	100	20	24	47
Vanilla Wafers, Nabisco	100	73	5	16
2 cookies	6	4	0	1
4 cookies	14	10	1	2
Wheat Thins	100	63	7	25
5 crackers	9	6	1	2
Zwiebach	100	74	12	9
1 piece	7	5	1	1

PROTEIN FOODS

1. CHEESE

Household Measurement	Gram Weight	C	P	F
American	100	2	22	30
Blue Mold	100	2	22	31
1 oz.	28	1	6	9
Camembert	100	2	18	25
1 oz.	28	1	5	7
Cheddar	100	2	25	32
1 tbsp. grated	7	0	2	2
1 oz.	28	1	7	9
Cottage, Creamed	100	3	14	4
1 oz.	28	1	4	1
Cream	100	2	8	38
1 oz.	28	1	2	11
Old English	100	2	31	30
1 oz.	28	1	6	8

(1 Cont.) Household Measurement	Gram Weight	C	P	F
Parmesan	100	3	36	26
1 oz.	28	1	10	7
Roquefort	100	2	22	31
1 oz.	28	1	6	9
Swiss	100	2	26	27
1 oz.	28	1	7	8
Velveeta	100	10	18	25
1 oz.	28	3	5	7

2. DAIRY PRODUCTS

Household Measurement	Gram Weight	C	P	F
Butter	100	0	0	80
1 cup	224	1	1	180
1 tbsp.	15	0	0	12
Cream				
Coffee Cream	100	4	3	20
1 tbsp.	15	1	0	3
Half and Half	100	5	3	12
1 tbsp.	15	1	0	2
Dream Whip	100	30	9	58
1 tbsp., prepared		1	0	1
Sour	100	3	2	18
1 oz. or 2 tbsp.	30	1	1	5
Whipping	100	4	3	31
1 tbsp.	15	0	0	5
Ice Cream				
Standard Vanilla	100	21	4	12
1 average scoop	75	16	3	9
Standard Ice Milk	100	23	5	5
Sherbet	100	31	1	1
Carnation Slender Frozen Dessert	100	25	5	5
Darigold Sugar Free	100	20	3	10
Darigold Trim	100	23	5	5
Milk				
Whole Milk	100	5	3	4
1 cup	240	12	7	10
2% Milk	100	5	3	2
1 cup	240	12	7	5

(2 Cont.) Household Measurement	Gram Weight	C	P	F
Skim Milk	100	5	3	0
1 cup	240	12	7	0
Whole Milk, dry powder	100	38	26	28
1 tbsp.	7	3	2	2
Skim Milk, dry powder	100	52	36	0
1 tbsp.	7	4	3	0
Evaporated Milk	100	10	7	8
1 tbsp.	16	2	1	1
1/2 cup	126	13	9	10
Buttermilk	100	5	3	0
1 cup	240	12	7	0
Yogurt (unflavored — from partially skimmed milk)	100	5	3	2
1 cup	240	12	7	5

3. EGGS

Household Measurement	Gram Weight	C	P	F
Egg (whole), 2	100	0	12	12
1 large egg	50	0	6	6
Egg, white	100	0	11	0
1 egg white	30	0	3	0
Egg, yolk	100	0	16	31
1 egg yolk	20	0	3	6

4. MEATS

Food values for 100 grams (edible portion) of meat cooked (broiled or baked), all fat removed.

	C	P	F
Low Fat Meats	0	30	6

Ham, Lamb, Beef, Pork, or Veal

Round steaks	Sirloin
Rump roasts	Dried meat
Flank steaks	Leg roast

	C	P	F
Medium Fat Meats	0	30	10

Ham, Lamb, Beef, Pork, or Veal

Rib roasts	Club steaks
Rib steaks	Shoulder roasts
Lean ground beef	Loin roasts
Porter house	Loin chops
T-bone steaks	

(4 Cont.)	C	P	F
High Fat Meats			
Hamburger	0	24	20
Any cut of meat heavily marbled with fat	0	24	20
Spare ribs	0	21	39
Liver	3	29	4
Sausage and Cold Cuts			
Bacon	3	30	52
Bockwurst	1	11	24
Bologna	1	12	27
Canadian Bacon	0	28	18
Country-style Sausage	0	15	31
Frankfurters	2	14	20
Liverwurst	2	15	27
Boiled Ham	0	19	17
Minced Ham	4	14	17
Pork Sausage, links	0	18	44
Salami	1	18	26
Venison	0	34	6

5. FISH

Food values for 100 grams of edible fish, cooked (broiled or baked) unless otherwise specified.

	C	P	F
Abalone, canned	2	16	0
Clams, raw	2	13	2
Clams, canned	2	16	3
Cod, canned	0	19	0
Cod, cooked	0	29	5
Crab, cooked or canned	1	17	2
Fish Sticks, frozen and cooked	7	17	9
Halibut	0	25	7
Lobster, canned or cooked	0	19	2
Oysters, canned	5	9	2
Oysters, cooked (fried)	19	9	14
Red Snapper, raw	0	20	1
Salmon, cooked	0	27	7
canned, Chinook	0	20	14
canned, all others	0	20	9
Sardines (canned in oil)	2	19	12
Scallops, cooked	0	23	1
Scallops, frozen and fried	11	18	8

(5 Cont.)	C	P	F
Shrimps, canned	0	24	1
Shrimps, French fried	10	20	11
Smelt	0	15	6
Sole or Flounder	0	30	8
Trout	0	24	15
Tuna, canned in oil	0	29	8
Tuna, canned in water	0	30	2

6. POULTRY

Food values for 100 grams of cooked poultry, edible portions.

	C	P	F
Chicken			
Broiled	0	24	4
Fryers	3	30	12
Roasted	0	30	9
Canned	0	22	12
Duck			
Roasted	0	30	10
Goose			
Roasted	0	34	10
Turkey			
Roasted	0	30	8

FAT FOODS

	Household Measurement	Gram Weight	C	P	F
Butter, Oleomargarine		100	0	0	80
	1 tsp.	5	0	0	4
	1 tbsp.	15	0	0	12
Cream (See Dairy Products)					
Lard, shortening		100	0	0	100
	1 tbsp.	15	0	0	15
	1 cup	220	0	0	220
Oils, corn, olive, etc.		100	0	0	100
	1 tbsp.	15	0	0	15
Mayonnaise		100	2	1	80
	1 tbsp.	15	0	0	13
Salad Dressing (mayonnaise type)		100	14	1	42
	1 tbsp.	15	2	0	6

(FAT FOODS Cont.)

Household Measurement	Gram Weight	C	P	F
French Dressing	100	17	1	39
1 tbsp.	15	3	0	6
Thousand Island Dressing	100	15	1	50
1 tbsp.	15	2	0	8
Roquefort Dressing	100	7	5	52
1 tbsp.	15	1	1	8
Olives, green	100	0	1	13
2 olives	10	0	0	1
Olives, ripe	100	2	1	20
2 olives	10	0	0	2

NUTS

Household Measurement	Gram Weight	C	P	F
Almonds, shelled	100	20	17	54
12 to 15 nuts	15	3	3	9
Brazil nuts, shelled	100	9	14	67
4 medium nuts	15	1	2	10
Cashews, roasted	100	28	17	46
6 to 8 nuts	15	4	3	7
Coconut, shredded, dried	100	23	7	65
1 cup	62	12	4	40
Coconut, fresh	100	9	4	35
Macadamia nuts	100	13	8	72
6 nuts	15	2	1	11
Peanuts, roasted	100	16	26	50
1 tbsp. nuts	15	2	4	8
Peanut Butter	100	18	26	49
1 tbsp.	15	3	4	7
Pecans, shelled	100	12	9	71
12 halves	15	2	1	11
Planters, dry roasted peanuts	100	21	27	44
Walnuts	100	14	15	64
8 to 15 halves	15	2	2	10

SOUPS

Soup (undiluted) food values for 100 grams. 100 grams is approximately 1/3 of a can before milk or water is added.

	C	P	F
Campbell's			
Asparagus	9	2	3
Bean with Bacon	16	7	4
Beef	9	8	2
Beef Noodle	7	3	2
Cheddar Cheese	8	5	10
Chili Beef	13	6	4
Cream of Celery	6	1	4
Cream of Chicken	7	3	6
Cream of Mushroom	7	2	9
Cream of Potato	9	1	2
Cream of Vegetable	8	2	5
Chicken Gumbo	8	2	1
Chicken Noodle	7	3	1
Chicken Vegetable	8	3	2
Chicken with Rice	5	3	1
Chicken and Stars	6	3	1
Clam Chowder, Boston and Manhattan	9	2	2
Green Pea	19	7	2
Minestrone	8	5	3
Noodles and Ground Beef	8	4	4
Onion	3	4	1
Oyster Stew	5	2	3
Split Pea w/Ham	19	8	2
Tomato	12	1	2
Tomato Rice	15	1	2
Turkey Noodle	7	3	3
Vegetable	9	3	2
Vegetable Beef	5	6	2
Vegetable, Old Fashioned	10	2	2
Campbell's Chunky Soups (Do Not Dilute)			
per 1/2 can			
Chunky Beef	21	15	7
Chunky Chicken	20	14	7
Chunky Sirloin Burger	21	12	7
Chunky Turkey	17	11	5
Snow's			
Clam Chowder	10	5	2
Lipton Onion Soup Mix			
One package dry — 45 grams	21	6	3

MISCELLANEOUS FOODS

	Household Measurement	Gram Weight	C	P	F
Carbonated Beverages					
Ginger Ale	. . . .	100	8	0	0
Average, all others	. . . .	100	12	0	0
Carnation Instant Breakfast,					
1 envelope, dry	. . . .		24	7	0
1 serving with whole milk	. . . .		34	18	10
Chili Sauce	. . . .	100	24	3	0
1 tbsp.	. . . .	17	4	1	0
Chocolate, bitter	. . . .	100	29	6	53
1 square	. . . .	28	8	2	15
Cider	. . . .	100	12	1	0
Cocoa, dry powder	. . . .	100	49	8	24
Gelatin, unsweetened, dry	. . . .	100	0	85	0
1 envelope, Knox	. . . .	8	0	7	0
Gelatin, sweetened	. . . .	100	14	2	0
Ketchup	. . . .	100	25	2	0
1 tbsp.	. . . .	17	4	0	0
Meritene, dry powder	. . . .	100	58	33	0
4 tbsp.	. . . .	32	19	11	0
1 serving with whole milk	. . . .		32	18	10
Metrecal	. . . .	100	12	8	2
One 8 oz. can	. . . .	240	28	18	5
Ovaltine (plain)					
1 serving with whole milk	. . . .		22	11	10
Postum	. . . .	100	85	6	0
1 tsp.	. . . .	1	1	0	0
Soy Sauce	. . . .	100	10	6	1
1 tbsp.	. . . .	15	2	0	0
Worcestershire	. . . .	100	19	2	0
1 tbsp.	. . . .	15	3	0	0

PREPARED FOODS

	Gram Weight	C	P	F
Chun King				
Chicken Divider-Pak Chow Mein . . .	100	9	5	1
Beef Divider-Pak Chow Mein	100	8	6	2
Meatless Chow Mein	100	6	1	0

(PREPARED FOODS Cont.)

Household Measurement	Gram Weight	C	P	F
Subgum Chicken Chow Mein	100	6	2	0
Beef Chop Suey	100	5	3	1
Chicken Chow Mein	100	6	2	0
Chinese Vegetables	100	1	2	0
Chop Suey Vegetables	100	1	1	0
Nalley's				
Chili	100	12	8	8
Beef Stew	100	8	5	5
Lima Beans and Ham	100	13	7	4
Red Beans and Chili Gravy	100	16	6	2
Spaghetti and Meat	100	13	4	3
IXL Lasagne	100	12	4	3
IXL Chicken Ravioli	100	36	4	4
Potato Salad	100	18	2	9
Franco-American				
Beef Gravy	100	5	2	1
Chicken Gravy	100	5	2	6
Italian Style Spaghetti	100	14	4	1
Macaroni and Cheese	100	11	4	4
Spaghetti and Ground Beef	100	11	5	6
Spaghetti with Tomato Sauce	100	15	3	1
Heinz				
Beef Stew	100	6	6	4
Chicken Noodle Dinner	100	7	4	4
Chile Con Carne with Beans	100	11	8	6
Macaroni with Cheese Sauce	100	11	4	4
Spaghetti with Tomato Sauce & Cheese	100	16	2	2
Campbell Soup Co. (Swanson)				
Beef Meat Pie (8 oz.)	227	36	17	25
Beef T.V. Dinner	319	32	34	17
Chicken Meat Pie (8 oz.)	227	50	16	26
Fish 'n French Fries	276	40	26	18
Fried Shrimp T.V. Dinner	213	40	18	13
Fried Chicken T.V. Dinner	340	45	37	29
Swiss Steak T.V. Dinner	326	37	30	9
Turkey T.V. Dinner	347	42	29	13
Swift and Company				
Tamales with Sauce	100	15	4	7

FOOD SUBSTITUTES FOR A CALCULATED DIET

If your menu calls for 100 grams of a 12% Fruit, you can substitute one of the following:

100 grams of a 12% Fruit equals:
  200 grams of a   6% Fruit   66 grams of a 18% Fruit
  135 grams of a   9% Fruit   52 grams of Banana
   80 grams of a 15% Fruit

If your menu calls for an 18% Vegetable, you can substitute with one food from list below:

100 grams of an 18% Vegetable equals:
  90 grams of a 20% Vegetable
  80 grams of spaghetti, noodles, macaroni or rice
  34 grams of bread

If your menu calls for 30 grams of bread, you can substitute with one food from list below:

30 grams of bread equals:
  70 grams of rice, macaroni,   80 grams of a 20% Vegetable
    spaghetti, or noodles   90 grams of a 18% Vegetable

If your menu calls for 100 grams of a 9% Vegetable, you can substitute with one food from list below:

100 grams of a 9% Vegetable equals:
  150 grams of a 6% Vegetable   75 grams of a 12% Vegetable

Chapter 4 THE EXCHANGE DIET

GENERAL RULES FOR DIABETIC EXCHANGE DIET

1. Weigh or measure your food for the first three months, at least, to become familiar with proportions.

2. If your doctor has specified a Weighed Diet, use a gram scale. The gram weight listed for each food is the amount allowed for one serving or exchange.

3. If your doctor has specified a Household Measurement Diet, use a standard 8-ounce measuring cup and a measuring teaspoon or a measuring tablespoon. All measurements are level. The household measure is listed for each food in the food exchange lists and equals the amount allowed for one serving or exchange.

4. Food should be weighed or measured after cooking.

5. Eat only the foods on the diet list, and only in the amount specified.

6. Do not miss meals or eat between meals unless a snack has been prescribed by your doctor.

7. Eat meals at the same times each day.

8. Foods in each exchange list are interchangeable. When used in amounts specified they provide approximately the same amounts of carbohydrate, protein, and fat.

FREE FOODS: Allowed any time during day.

Noncaloric sweeteners, fat-free broth or bouillon, coffee, tea, dietetic carbonated beverages (sugar-free), horseradish, mustard, spices, herbs, vinegar and D-Zerta gelatin.

FOODS TO AVOID

Sugar, honey, candy, fruit canned with sugar, jam, jelly, syrup; all desserts; scalloped, creamed, or fried foods; and all alcoholic beverages.

EXCHANGE LISTS

---

1. VEGETABLE EXCHANGES — A

These vegetables are insignificant in carbohydrates, when raw may have 150 grams or 1 cup. When cooked, limit serving to 100 grams or 1/2 cup. (See listing on next page.)

(1 Cont.)

Asparagus	Dill pickles	Romaine
Bamboo shoots	Eggplant	Rhubarb
Beans	Greens	Sauerkraut
— green, snap, wax	— beet, chard, etc.	spinach
Broccoli	Lettuce	Squash, summer
Cabbage	Mushrooms	Tomato*
Cauliflower	Parsley	Tomato juice*
Celery	Peppers, green	V-8 Vegetable juice*
Chives	Pimento	Water cress
Cucumber	Radishes	Zucchini

*Limit serving to 100 grams or 1/2 cup.

2. VEGETABLE EXCHANGES — B

Each serving contains 7 grams of carbohydrate, 3 grams of protein.

Food	Gram Weight	Household Measurement
Artichokes, globe or French	75	1/2 cup
Bean sprouts	75	1 cup
Beets	75	1/2 cup
Brussel sprouts	100	2/3 cup
Carrots, raw	75	1 medium
Carrots, cooked, canned or frozen	100	2/3 cup
Hominy	50	1/3 cup
Leeks	75	3 (5" long)
Lima beans, canned	50	1/3 cup
Mixed frozen vegetables	50	1/3 cup
Onions, raw	75	1 medium
Onions, cooked, canned	100	1/2 cup
Okra	100	8-9 pods
Parsnips	55	1/4 cup
Peas, canned	50	1/4 cup
Peas, fresh or frozen	75	1/3 cup
Pumpkin	100	1/2 cup
Rutabagas	100	1/2 cup
Squash, winter baked	50	1/4 cup
Squash, winter boiled	100	1/2 cup
Turnips	100	2/3 cup

3. FRUIT EXCHANGES

Each serving contains 10 grams of carbohydrate, 1 gram of protein. Fruit should be fresh or waterpacked (W.P.) with or without artificial sweetening. Do not use commercially frozen fruit unless label says no sugar added.

Food	Gram Weight	Household Measurement
Apple (2" diameter)	80	1 small (1/2 med.)
Apple juice	80	1/3 cup
Applesauce	100	1/2 cup
Apricots, dried	15	3 halves
Apricots, fresh	85	2 medium
Apricot, nectar	75	1/3 cup
Apricots, stewed	50	2-3 halves
Apricots, W.P.	115	3 medium
Banana	50	1/2 small
Blackberries, fresh	115	3/4 cup
Blackberries, W.P.	170	1 cup
Blueberries	75	1/2 cup
Boysenberries	115	3/4 cup
Cantaloupe (5" diameter)	150	- 1/4
Cherries, sweet	55	1/3 c. (8 lge.)
Cherries, W.P.	85	1/2 cup
Cranberry juice, lo-calorie	200	scant 1 c.
Cranapple, lo-calorie	250	1 cup
Dates	15	2 to 3
Figs, dried	15	2 small
Figs, fresh	50	1 large
Figs, W.P.	85	3 medium
Fruit cocktail, W.P.	115	1/2 cup
Grapefruit, fresh	100	1/2 small
Grapefruit juice	115	1/2 cup
Grapefruit, W.P.	150	3/4 cup
Grapes	75	16 grapes
Grape juice	55	1/4 cup
Honeydew melon (7" diameter)	150	1/2 melon
Huckleberries	75	1/2 cup
Jello	70	1/3 cup
Lemon juice	120	1/2 cup
Lime juice	120	1/2 cup
Loganberries	85	1/2 cup

(3 Cont.)	Gram Weight	Household Measurement
Mango	70	1/2 small
Orange	85	1 small
Orange juice	100	1/2 cup
Oranges, mandarin, W.P.	170	2/3 cup
Papaya	115	1/3 medium
Peaches, fresh	115	1 medium
Peach nectar	85	1/3 cup
Peaches, W.P.	125	2/3 cup
Pears, fresh	75	1/2 small
Pear, nectar	85	1/3 cup
Pears, W.P.	125	2/3 cup
Pineapple, fresh	85	1 slice
Pineapple juice	85	1/3 slice
Pineapple, W.P.	100	1 slice
Plums, fresh	85	1½ medium
Plums, purple	55	1 medium
Plums, W.P.	100	2 medium
Prunes, dried	15	2
Prune juice	55	1/4 cup
Raspberries, fresh	115	3/4 cup
Raisins	15	1/8 cup
Rhubarb, raw cubed	250	2½ cups
Sherbet	35	1/2 scoop
Strawberries	150	1 cup
Tangerines	85	1 medium
Watermelon	170	1 cup

4. BREAD AND VEGETABLE EXCHANGES

Each serving contains 15 grams of carbohydrate, 3 grams of protein.

Food	Gram Weight	Household Measurement
BREADS		
Whole wheat, white, rye, etc.	28	1 slice
Bagel (average)	25	1/2 bagel
Baking powder biscuit*	35	1
Cornbread, unsweetened	35	1½" cube
Diet breads	23	2 slices
Doughnut, cake type plain*	32	1 average
English muffin	25	1/2 muffin

(4 Cont.)	Gram Weight	Household Measurement
Melba toast......................	20	5 pieces
Muffin (2" diameter)*..............	35	1
Roll, frankfurter...................	25	1/2 roll
Roll, hamburger...................	25	1/2 roll
Roll, soft dinner..................	30	1
Pancakes.........................	45	1-4"
Waffles, frozen*..................	48	1 rnd. or 2 sq.

CEREALS

	Gram Weight	Household Measurement
Cooked.........................	140	1/2 cup
Dry		
flakes..........................	25	1/2 cup
puffed..........................	20	1 cup
grape nuts.....................	17	1/8 cup

COOKIES AND CRACKERS

	Gram Weight	Household Measurement
Animal (Nabisco)..................	20	7
Angelfood cake..................	30	1 ounce
Arrowroot (Sunshine)..............	20	5
Ginger Snaps....................	18	6 cookies
Graham (Nabisco).................	20	3
Lorna Doone Cookies (Nabisco).......	23	3 cookies
Matzoth, round..................	15	3/4
Oyster crackers (Nabisco)...........	20	25 crackers
Popcorn.........................	20	1½ cups
Pretzels (Nabisco 3-Ring)...........	19	6 pretzels
Ritz (Nabisco)....................	25	8 crackers
Ry-Krisp.........................	20	3 crackers
Saltines (Nabisco).................	22	7 crackers
Wheat Thins (Nabisco)..............	20	12 crackers
Vanilla wafers....................	22	6 cookies
Zweibach.......................	21	3 pieces

FLOUR PRODUCTS

	Gram Weight	Household Measurement
Bisquick.........................	25	1/4 cup
Cornstarch......................	16	2 tbsp.
Flour...........................	20	2½ tbsp.
Macaroni, cooked.................	100	1/2 cup
Noodles, cooked..................	100	1/2 cup
Spaghetti, cooked.................	100	1/2 cup
Rice...........................	100	1/2 cup

(4 Cont.)	Gram Weight	Household Measurement
VEGETABLES		
Beans, cooked		
Baked beans	75	1/4 cup
Kidney beans, canned	95	1/2 cup
Kidney beans, dried, cooked	75	1/3 cup
Lima beans, frozen	85	1/3 cup
Lima beans, dried and cooked	70	1/3 cup
Corn, canned, fresh	80	1/2 cup
Corn, fresh, cob	80	1/3 ear
Garbanzos, cooked	75	1/8 cup
Jerusalem artichoke	85	1 medium
Peas, dry, split, cooked	75	1/3 cup
Potatoes, sweet	60	1/2 small
Potatoes, white	85	1 small
Potato chips**	30	15 chips
Potatoes, French fried*	40	8 pieces
Ice cream**	70	scant 1/2 cup
Ice milk*	70	scant 1/2 cup
Meritine, powdered, dry	25	3 tbsp.

*Omit 1 fat exchange
**Omit 2 fat exchanges

5. MEAT EXCHANGES (Protein Foods)
Each serving contains 9 grams of protein and 3 grams of fat. Weight is for edible portion only — remove all fat and bone.

Food	Gram Weight	Household Measurement
Meat and poultry (lean)		
Beef, lamb, ham, chicken, pork,		
turkey, liver	30	1 ounce
Cold cuts*	45	1 slice
Hot dogs*	60	1
Sausage**	60	2 links
Hamburger*	30	1 ounce

Fish
  Cod, halibut, salmon, tuna, clams,
  crab, lobster, red snapper,

(5 Cont.)	Gram Weight	Household Measurement
shrimp, sardines, scallops, smelt, trout	30	1 ounce
Bacon***	30	3 strips
Cheese		
Cheddar*	30	1 ounce
Cottage, creamed	65	1/4 cup
Parmesan*	30	1 ounce
Roquefort*	30	1 ounce
Swiss*	30	1 ounce
Velveeta*	50	1¾ oz.
Egg	50	1 lge. or 2 sm.
Peanut butter**	30	2-3 tbsp.

*Omit one fat exchange
**Omit two fat exchanges
***Omit three fat exchanges

(As bacon is very high in fat, it is suggested that it be used from the fat list, rather than the meat list.

6. FAT EXCHANGES

Each serving contains 5 grams of fat.

Food	Gram Weight	Household Measurement
Avocado	30	1/4 medium
Bacon	10	1 strip
Butter or margarine	5	1 tsp.
Cream, heavy	15	1 tbsp.
Cream, light (half and half)	25	2 tbsp.
Cream, sour	15	1 tbsp.
Cream cheese	15	1 tbsp.
French dressing	15	1 tbsp.
Mayonnaise	5	1 tsp.
Oil or shortening	5	1 tsp.
Nuts	10	6 small
Olives	30	8 small
Salad Dressing (mayonnaise type)	15	1 tbsp.

7. MILK EXCHANGES

Each serving contains 12 grams of carbohydrate, 7 grams of protein and from 0-10 grams of fat. The (*) stars indicate the amount of fat in each item.** = 10 grams of fat or 2 fat exchanges. * = 5 grams of fat or 1 fat exchange. 0 stars indicates no fat or skim milk. Usually the diet plan will be made out to include the specific type of milk used in the diet. Please check with the dietitian regarding your diet.

Food	Gram Weight	Household Measurement
Milk, whole**	240	1 cup
Milk, 2%*	240	1 cup
Milk, skim	240	1 cup
Milk, evaporated**	120	1/2 cup
Milk, dry powder skim	30	2 tbsp.
Buttermilk	240	1 cup
Yogurt, unflavored*	240	1 cup
Ice cream**	55	1/3 cup
Ice milk*	55	1/3 cup

8. SOUP EXCHANGES

The value of each exchange is carbohydrate 9 grams, protein 3 grams, fat 3 grams, per exchange in grams weight noted below. Gram 100 equals approximately 1/3 of can. Measure before adding water.

	Gram Weight	Household Measurement
Campbell's		
Asparagus	100	1/2 cup
Bean with Bacon	50	1/3 cup
Beef...........................	100	1/2 cup
Beef Noodle	140	2/3 cup
Cheddar Cheese	120	1/2 cup
Chicken Vegetable	120	1/2 cup
Chili Beef	70	1/3 cup
Chicken Gumbo	120	1/2 cup
Chicken Noodle.................	125	1/2 cup
Chicken with Rice	175	7/8 cup
Chicken and Stars	150	2/3 cup
Clam Chowder	100	1/2 cup

(8 Cont.)	Gram Weight	Household Measurement
Clam Chowder, Manhattan	100	1/2 cup
Cream of Celery	150	2/3 cup
Cream of Chicken	140	2/3 cup
Cream of Mushroom	140	2/3 cup
Cream of Potato	100	1/2 cup
Cream of Vegetable	100	1/2 cup
Green Pea	50	1/4 cup
Minestrone	120	1/2 cup
Noodles and Ground Beef	120	1/2 cup
Onion	200	1 cup
Oyster Stew	300	1¼ cups
Split Pea with Ham	50	1/4 cup
Tomato	85	1/3 cup
Tomato Rice	70	1/3 cup
Turkey Noodle	120	1/2 cup
Vegetable	100	1/2 cup
Vegetable Beef	150	2/3 cup
Vegetable, Old Fashioned	100	1/2 cup
Snow's Clam Chowder	100	1/2 cup
Lipton's Onion Soup Mix	45	1/2 pkg.-dry
Chunky Soups (Do Not Dilute)		
Chunky Beef	140	2/3 cup
Chunky Chicken	140	2/3 cup
Chunky Sirloin Burger	140	2/3 cup
Chunky Turkey	140	2/3 cup

Chapter 5   ADDITIONAL DIETARY INFORMATION

VITAMINS
Some important facts:

1. Vitamins are essential to good health, to use of carbohydrates, proteins and fats for energy, and for formation of tissues and certain essential substances (enzymes).

2. Recommended daily allowances are sufficient to prevent deficiency diseases and are supplied in a diet containing adequate amounts of the four food groups (cereals, meats, fruits and vegetables). However, vitamin D daily requirements are not met unless there is adequate exposure to sunlight or unless vitamin D is part of diet. These daily vitamin needs are greater during pregnancy and lactation.

3. Caution is necessary when taking supplementary vitamin A and D as both can have adverse effects if taken in excess.

4. Foods should be cooked lightly, in small amounts of water.

Table 2 lists the various vitamins, their actions and food sources. Under normal circumstances a well structured diet will result in an adequate intake of vitamins.

VEGETARIAN DIETS

In a 1973 issue of *THE MEDICAL LETTER* on Drugs and Therapeutics*, vegetarian diets were discussed because of the increasing numbers of people using such diets. Some people are vegans or complete vegetarians. Others called lacto-vegetarians include in their diet, milk, butter and cheese. Another group, lacto-ovo-vegetarians, also eat eggs. Complete vegetarians may lack essential amino acids present in certain proteins and vitamin B12. Those who drink cow's milk can prevent such deficiencies. Cereals, soybeans peas, beans and lentils are a source of some of the essential amino acids. Therefore, the vegetarian should carefully plan the inclusion of as many of the above-noted foods in diet planning as possible. If a complete vegetarian diet is followed, it would be advisable to take a vitamin B12 tablet daily to prevent the appearance of a macrocytic anemia.

*The Medical Letter 15:30, March 30, 1973

TABLE 2.

VITAMINS: ACTIONS AND SOURCES

Vitamin Recommended Daily Allowances of		Actions	Food Sources
A	1.4 Children 2-4000 Adults 5000	Important to the function of photo-sensitive parts of the eye (i.e. Retina) and aids in vision in dim light. Involved in action of vitamin E, and function of the conjunctiva, the outer covering of the eye, mucous membranes and skin.	Deep yellow vegetables, deep-green leafy vegetables, fruits. Liver, kidney, whole milk, eggs, fish.
B_1 Thiamine	1.5 mg.	Involved in metabolism of carbohydrates.	Whole grain bread, cereals, flour, meats, poultry, fish, milk, green vegetables, nuts, legumes.
B_2 Riboflavin	1.5 mg.	Aids in body cell use of hydrogen.	Organ meats, milk, eggs, green leafy vegetables.
B_3 Niacin	20.0 mg.	Promotes energy production in body cells.	Whole grain cereals, enriched bread, flour, meats, poultry, fish, nuts, legumes.
B_6 Pyridoxine	2.0 mg.	Involved in protein metabolism and function of nerve cells.	Meat, poultry, fish, vegetables, potatoes, eggs, bananas.
Pantothenic Acid	?	Assists energy metabolism, fat and cholesterol synthesis.	Meat, poultry, fish, whole grain cereals, legumes, some in fruit, vegetables, milk
B_{12} Cobalamin	4 mcg.	Aids in formation mature red blood cells, and DNA and RNA.	Organ meats, muscle meats, fish, poultry, eggs, milk, cheese.
Folic Acid	400 mcg.	Aids in formation mature red blood cells.	Organ meats, muscle meats, poultry, fish, whole grain cereals, eggs, apricots, deep-green leafy vegetables.
C Ascorbic Acid	60 mg.	Assists in use of folic acid, and formation of bone, teeth, blood vessels and assists in wound healing.	Citrous fruits, tomatoes, melons, strawberries, fresh potatoes, green leafy vegetables, cabbage, broccoli.
D	400-I.U.	Aids in absorption of calcium in diet — and works with parathyroid hormone and calcitonin to control concentration calcium in blood plasma, bone, etc.	Vit D enriched milk
E Tocopherol	15-20 mg.	Involved in maintenance of reproductive system of certain rodents — (not shown in men) may assist function of muscle and stability of red blood cells.	Vegetable and seed oils

ALCOHOL AND D.M.

Much controversy surrounds the use of alcohol. Philosophical comments will be limited to the following. (1) It is accepted that excessive use of alcohol can be detrimental to one's health. (2) Alcohol may lead to difficulty in arriving at a diagnosis of hypoglycemia. (See p. 100). (3) Consumption of alcohol may add greatly to the daily intake of calories.

The ingestion of alcohol is quickly followed by a rise in blood alcohol content. It is then distributed throughout many body tissues, particularly the liver and kidneys where it is oxidized to carbon dioxide. This process furnishes considerable energy for the body, i.e. seven calories per gram, or 210 calories per ounce. Although alcohol is not converted into sugar, it provides calories and thereby leads to weight gain.

Alcohol can prime the output of insulin of normally functioning cells. It can also suppress in some persons the action of epinephrine and the conversion of protein to sugar — mechanisms that protect from hypoglycemia. Some patients receiving one of the sulfonylurea oral tablets for the treatment of diabetes may have an unusual reaction to alcohol. This consists of a flushing and warmth of the face, a pounding headache, dizziness, and nausea lasting for nearly an hour (antabuse effect). For these reasons, and for the more serious effects of chronic alcohol-

FOOD VALUE OF COMMON ALCOHOLIC BEVERAGES

Drink	Measure	Total Grams	Grams Alcohol	Grams CHO	Calories
Ale, beer, stout	1 glass (8 oz.)	240	7-14	7-14	80-150
Brandy, Gin, Rum	1 oz.	30	10-13	—	75- 90
Cordials, liqueurs	1 oz. jigger	30	6- 9	6-13	65-100
Wines, sweet	3½ oz.	100	13-15	8-14	140-165
dry	glass	100	10-11	1- 4	110-175
Whiskey Bourbon, Irish Rye, Scotch	1 oz. jigger	30	11-12	—	75- 85

ism, there is no good reason for the use of alcohol. However, since certain people will use alcohol, they should do so with caution and awareness. Cocktails should use either water or sugarless carbonated beverages as a dilutant; better yet as a substitute. If food is consumed during the social hour, some reduction of food may be desirable at the following meal. Ingestion of food during or shortly after the taking of more than one drink of alcohol will help to avoid hypoglycemia.

CALCULATION OF CALORIES FROM ALCOHOL:

1 ml. alcohol contributes 7 calories.

30 ml. (1 oz.) alcohol contributes 210 calories.

100 proof whiskey is 50 percent alcohol.

30 ml. would contribute 105 calories.

1 ml. alcohol (800 mg.) per kilogram body weight, or 70 ml. to be ingested by someone weighing 154 pounds (70 kg.) within one hour, would raise the blood level in two hours to 10 mg. per 100 ml. of blood, i.e. a level of 0.10 percent. A blood level in excess of 0.10 percent is established by law in some states as evidence of intoxication. It is illegal to drive an automobile with this blood alcohol level.

DIETARY FAT AND ARTERIOSCLEROSIS

Since there is evidence of some relationship between dietary fat and thickening of arteries, it is best to have some guidelines about which foods might best be avoided, particularly by those who may be advised to make such changes.

It is probable that arteriosclerosis is influenced by two aspects of dietary fat: first, the percentage of total calories provided as fat, and, secondly, the relative proportion of "saturated" and "polyunsaturated" fat. At our present state of knowledge, it is probably wise to attempt both a decrease in the total fat in the diet and to increase the relative proportion of polyunsaturated to saturated fat. The degree of saturation of fat corresponds roughly with the melting point of the fat, fats which tend to remain solid at room temperature being more saturated than those fats which take a liquid form at room temperature.

The following general rules will result in a desirable ratio of polyunsaturated to saturated fat where such a diet seems indicated.

1. Not more than two eggs a week, however, egg white permitted.

2. Use skimmed or low fat milk. Avoid cheese except for "dry curd" cottage cheese.

3. Use fish or fowl for at least two-thirds of the meat courses throughout the week instead of ham, beef, pork or lamb. Cut all visible fat from ham, beef, pork or lamb. Do not use bacon.

4. Use spreads especially prepared with a high percentage of polyunsaturated fats.

5. Avoid foods containing chocolate.

6. Use corn oil, soybean or cottonseed oil for cooking; avoid animal fat and bacon, butter, solid "hydrogenated" vegetable oils, lard, cream sauces and gravies.

7. The polyunsaturated fat content of the nut is variable, depending on the type of nut. In general, nuts other than the coconut contain a desirable proportion of polyunsaturated fat.

Under what circumstances is it important to lower the total fat content and increase the relative proportion of polyunsaturated fats in the diet? This question is difficult to answer at present. Some authorities feel that all would be better off if there was less use of saturated fats in the diet. Consideration should be given to controlling the dietary fat under the following circumstances:

1. Where there is existing evidence of arteriosclerosis involving the coronary arteries, particularly where this occurs at a relatively early age.

2. Where repeated fasting determinations have shown the blood lipids to be elevated above the normal range.

3. Where there is a strong family history of coronary heart disease, particularly where this has occurred before the age of 60.

4. Possibly in diabetes with onset under the age of forty.

Part 3

TREATMENT of DIABETES MELLITUS

Chapter 6   ORAL TREATMENT OF ADULT ONSET DM

ORAL TREATMENT OF ADULT-ONSET D.M.

Reference has been made to the use of oral medication for the treatment of adult onset diabetes. (See p. 23.) It was pointed out that the F.D.A. has issued warnings concerning their use. While many physicians support this action of the F.D.A., many other equally reputable physicians stand in opposition to it. The latter feel that where dietary efforts fail to control adult diabetes, there may be occasions for the use of one of these drugs in conjunction with dietary management.

CLASSES OF ORAL MEDICATIONS AND THEIR SIDE EFFECTS

1. Biquanides: DBI — Meltrol — Phenformin
    — TD capsules of 50 mg. and 100 mg. strength.
        The capsules are taken after meals in divided doses. The TD Capsule has longer activity than the short-acting tablet.
    — Tablet — 25 mg. size.

Side effects relate to larger doses and include nausea, loss of appetite, and occasionally diarrhea and weakness. A metallic taste may be noted. The medicine can be used in conjunction with insulin or the sulfonylureas. DBI is rarely a cause of hypoglycemia.

2. Sulfonylureas.
    Diabinese — 100 mg. and 250 mg. blue tablets
    Dymelor — 250 mg. white and 500 mg. yellow tablets
    Orinase —   500 mg white tablet
    Tolinase — 100 mg., 250 mg., 500 mg.

The sulfonylureas may act by increasing the responsiveness of the insulin-secreting cells of the pancrease to glucose and by suppressing glucagon production. The first preparation, Carbutamide or BZ55, was active against bacteria in the manner of the sulfa drugs. This is because the sulfonylureas are chemically related to the sulfa drugs. Carbutamide is no longer available in this country. The other preparations act in a manner similar to Carbutamide, but do not have any anti-bacterial activity. They differ in their durations of activity.
    — Orinase is short-acting and often is required in two or more daily doses. It is useful in adult onset diabetes, particularly in the elder-

ly, and in persons with a history of impaired kidney function.

— Dymelor can be conveniently taken in one or two doses daily. Because it has some diuretic action it may be selected for use in patients with heart disease.

— Tolinase is often prescribed in divided doses, and may be used by those with a history of heart failure.

— Diabinese is longer-acting than the above and can be given in a single daily dose. It is best to avoid its use where there are problems of fluid retention in the body.

The side effects in this group of medications most commonly are:

— Hypoglycemia

— Gastrointestinal — nausea, indigestion, loss of appetite, diarrhea, rarely jaundice.

— Skin rashes, petachiae (i.e. minute bruises), increased sensitivity of the skin to sun.

— Blood, i.e., a drop in the white cell count.

— Peculiar reaction in some persons taking alcohol. (See p. 78).

Sulfonylureas are usually prescribed for those with adult onset diabetes who are not sufficiently well controlled by dietary measures.* At times it is more convenient for a patient with arthritis, tremors or paralysis to take one of the tablets rather than insulin. Sulfonylureas are not used in the treatment of juvenile diabetes, nor are they recommended for anyone showing ketones in the urine. Insulin is preferable in the course of severe infections. The F.D.A. cautions about their use during pregnancy.

HYPOGLYCEMIA AND TABLETS FOR ORAL TREATMENT OF D.M.

Sulfonylureas are capable of producing hypoglycemia. This effect may be prolonged and, therefore, such experiences should be reported to the physician or his nurse. In addition to the usual treatment for hypoglycemia, it may also be advisable to take supplementary or more substantial feedings.

If other medications are being used and one of the sulfonylurea drugs is prescribed, check with the prescribing physician about its use in conjunction with these other medications.

*See reference to F.D.A. warning regarding the use of oral anti-diabetic therapy and its possible contribution to coronary disease, page 23.

MEDICINE CAPABLE OF INCREASING THE RISK OF HYPO-GLYCEMIA WHEN USED WITH A SULFONYLUREA

Alcohol	Dilantin
Benemid	Salicylates
Butazolidin	Tandearil
Dicumarol (Coumadin)	Tranquilizers (certain)

Chapter 7 INSULIN TREATMENT OF DM

Since the dramatic introduction of insulin therapy in 1922, no spectacular improvements have been made in the management of insulin — dependent diabetes. Insulin therapy has been refined, however, through introduction of longer acting insulins, more highly purified insulin and recently U-100 insulin. U-100 insulin satisfies a long-time goal of the American Diabetes Association — simpler measurement and decreasing frequency of errors in dosage. The next dramatic advance in insulin therapy may come with the introduction of an implantable mechanical package which will not only be able to detect a rise in blood glucose, but through a miniaturized electrical system, cause the release of a burst of insulin from a reservoir.* This is the response of insulin-secreting cells of the pancreas.[1,2] Another exciting possibility being evaluated is beta-cell transplant. These cells are cultured (grown) to provide a sufficient number for use. Hopefully the cells will be developed such that they will not trigger rejection mechanisms in the host. This would make it unnecessary for the host to be given immuno-suppressive drugs. Transplanted beta-cells have been shown to work, secreting insulin in response to an increase of blood glucose.[3,4,5]

INDIVIDUAL REACTIONS TO THE USE OF INSULIN

Before any further explanation about the use of insulin it might be well to discuss the diabetic's reaction to the idea of taking insulin.

When sick for the first time with many of the severe symptoms of uncontrolled diabetes, many will feel relief to learn the symptoms can be controlled with insulin treatment. Others will marvel at how quickly

*For further information, see article — Soeldner, J. Stuart, Special Report: "Current Status of the Artificial Beta Cell and Implantation of Islets". A.D.A. Forecast, 26:1, July-August, 1973.

they improve once insulin injections are started. Most will recognize the unique value of insulin and quickly adjust to the need for daily injections of insulin.

An adult with a milder form of diabetes and only a few symptoms may either immediately accept the physician's recommendations or have some hesitancy about starting insulin. Doctors have heard patients remark, "You are never going to get me to take that — I can't stand the sight of a needle", while some elderly, even tremulous persons practice and practice to become proficient at insulin injection. Others have reacted, "But I would rather not take it — once I begin I will always have to take it". This is probably so. On the other hand, many adults show a gradual decrease in need for insulin and eventually have insulin injections discontinued.

Parents of some small children are initially distressed by their child's reluctance to be injected. When insulin administration is performed with some explanation and in a professional manner in the hospital environment, it usually becomes an accepted procedure. It is helpful if this same positive approach prevails at home. Hesitancy and uncertainty on the part of the parent may cause the child to respond in a similar fashion. The parent does not need to bribe the child nor show emotion at this time. There will be other occasions to show one's love and affection. With firmness, perserverance and supportive reassurances insulin injections will gradually become a routine procedure for both parent and child.

FACTS ABOUT INSULIN
INSULIN IS AVAILABLE IN THE FOLLOWING CONCENTRATIONS

1. U-40 and U-80 — the usual concentration used in past years.
2. U-100 — which will eventually replace U-40 and U-80 insulin.
3. U-500 — for unique cases requiring high doses of insulin.

When switching from U-40 to U-80 concentration of insulin many diabetics wonder if they are taking twice as much insulin. As there are 40 units of insulin in 1 ml. or 1 cc. of solution of U-40 insulin, as compared to 80 units in 1 ml. of U-80 insulin, it means that there are twice as many units of insulin in 1 ml. of U-80 insulin. IT DOES NOT MEAN THAT 1 UNIT OF U-80 INSULIN IS TWICE AS STRONG AS 1 UNIT OF U-40 INSULIN.

    1 unit of U-40 = 1 unit of U-80 = 1 unit of U-100 insulin
    10 units of U-40 = 10 units of U-80 = 10 units of U-100 insulin, and

whereas 10 units of U-40 insulin is in 1/4 ml. of solution, 10 units of U-80 insulin is in only 1/8 ml. and 10 units of U-100 insulin is placed in only 1/10 ml.

A unit of insulin is the quantity of insulin crystals which lowers the blood glucose in test animals by a specific amount.

INFORMATION ABOUT LILLY U-40, U-80, U-100 and U-500 SINGLE PEAK INSULINS, i.e. INSULINS OF IMPROVED PURITY

These insulins are highly purified during production by the removal of non-insulin protein materials. As a result, these insulins are:
1. More stable at room temperature.
2. Less likely to lead to insulin resistance.
3. Less likely to cause skin allergy.
4. Less likely to lead to insulin atrophy.

In fact, we already have good evidence that "single peak" mixed beef and pork insulin will effectively correct lipodystrophy when injected directly into the affected areas. Those which fail to improve may respond to either "single peak" or "single component" pork insulin.

There will be less opportunity for errors in insulin dose measurement when U-100 insulin and U-100 insulin syringes are universally used.

U-100 insulin is available in all of the various types used. The bottles are boldly marked in black on white, and the bottle caps are bright orange.

When using U-100 insulin, U-100 insulin syringes must also be used. The use of any other insulin syringe can result in dosage error. Both disposable and glass reusable syringes are available. The glass syringes are available in both the full 100 unit syringe, which is marked by 2 units, and a short 35 unit syringe, marked by 1 unit. The 35 unit syringe is more accurate for small doses of insulin.

Because U-100 insulin is a more concentrated insulin than either U-40 or U-80 insulin, patients use less volume. Therefore, some high dosage users are spared extra injections. A UNIT OF U-100 INSULIN IS AS POTENT AS A UNIT OF ANY OTHER STRENGTH OF THE SAME INSULIN, EVEN THOUGH THE VOLUME IS LESS.

For you to change from U-40 or U-80 to U-100 insulin:
1. Buy only U-100 insulin.

2. Buy only U-100 syringes.

3. Take the number of units of insulin your physician instructs you to take.

TYPES OF INSULIN FALL INTO THREE CLASSES:

1. Short acting insulin — duration of action is 6 to 8 hours.*
   Regular (crystalline zinc) insulin is clear, colorless insulin.

2. Intermediate acting insulin — duration of action for:
   Semilente insulin — 14 to 18 hours.
   Lente insulin —   20 to 26 hours.
   NPH insulin —   20 to 26 hours.

3. Long acting insulin — duration of action for:
   Ultralente —   36 or more hours.

Insulins other than regular are cloudy white in appearance. Graphs indicating the peak hours of and duration of each type of insulin are to be found in Fig. 9, page 98.

PREPARATION FOR INSULIN USE AT HOME

When purchasing insulin, always note the expiration date on the box. Be certain the insulin is used by this date, as the potency thereafter cannot be guaranteed. Occasionally druggists sell insulin at a reduced price when the expiration date is near. This insulin is safe when used before the expiration date.

TYPES OF INSULIN SYRINGES AND NEEDLES

There are many styles and types of syringes from which to choose. First, the diabetic should always ask his doctor which insulin concentration should be used, U-40, U-80 or U-100 insulin. He should then make certain the syringe matches the concentration of insulin being used. NEVER use more than one concentration of insulin or a double calibrated syringe (one with both U-40 and U-80 scales). The syringe with the double scale can too easily lead to error by measuring on the wrong scale.

---

*Not infrequently the actual response in insulin-dependent diabetics, who have taken insulin for two years or more is delayed. Therefore the peak action for regular insulin may be as late as 6 hours and the duration of action as long as 10 to 12 hours. (Doctors R. Bressler and J. Galloway in NUTRITION TODAY, July/August 1971.)

Both plastic disposable syringes and glass reusable syringes are available. While plastic syringes are convenient, for the greatest accuracy, we continue to recommend the use of glass syringes. It may be difficult to clear air bubbles from the plastic syringes. Glass syringes cost more initially, but since they are able to be periodically sterilized and re-used, they may last for a long time. There are several styles of glass syringes, both long and short, in U-40, U-80, and U-100, 1 ml. and 2 ml. The cost begins at approximately $4.00. Many are using 1-cc. (100-unit) disposable syringes which have implanted needles 25G, 26G, either 1/2" or 5/8" in length.

Today disposable needles are the most widely used. Designed for one time use, they are individually packaged and pre-sterilized. Most of these needles have a plastic hub and a stainless steel shaft and are of excellent quality. As the length of the needle required is determined by the thickness of the fat layer, advice of the physician or nurse will help determine the best length for each individual. These needles are available in 1/2 inch, 5/8 inch, 7/8 inch, 1 inch or 1-1/2 inch lengths.

□ EQUIPMENT USED FOR INJECTION OF INSULIN

Syringe; Needles
Cotton balls
70% Isopropyl alcohol
Container for insulin syringe
Glass container for alcohol soaked cotton balls
Sterilizing equipment — Pan
                          Strainer

□ CARE OF NON-DISPOSABLE EQUIPMENT

1. Take syringe apart.
2. Wash thoroughly with soap and water.
   Use pipe cleaner to clean tip of syringe.
3. Rinse in clear running water.
   Place in strainer.
4. Place strainer with equipment in pan of clean water covering equipment.
5. Put pan on stove — bring water to boil.
   Boil 15 minutes.
6. Remove strainer from pan. Empty pan.
7. Return strainer to pan. Allow to cool.
8. Remove container from strainer.
   Fill 1/2 full with 70% Isopropyl Alcohol.

9. Reassemble syringe by holding outside barrel between fingers and plunger top by fingers.
10. Use fresh needle.

RESTERILIZE EVERY 10 — 15 DAYS.

SUGGESTIONS FOR GLASS SYRINGES THAT DO NOT WORK SMOOTHLY

Patients sometimes complain that the glass syringe will stick together and not work smoothly. Usually the following procedure will combat this problem:

1. Take syringe apart and wash thoroughly with mild soap and warm water.

2. Rinse thoroughly.

3. Put a dab of glycerin on the tip of the plunger. Replace plunger in barrel portion of syringe and push up and down several times.

4. Take the syringe apart again and boil for 15 minutes in a pan of water to which 1 tablespoon of vinegar has been added.

5. Following a cooling period, put syringe together and place in alcohol container until ready to use.

It is usually helpful to re-boil the syringe in the vinegar water weekly, to prevent sticking.

INSTRUCTIONS FOR INSULIN ADMINISTRATION

Filling the syringe with insulin:

1. Wash hands.

2. Gather and assemble equipment: insulin, alcohol, cotton balls, syringe and needle.

3. Remove syringe and needle from the container and remove as much of the alcohol as possible by pulling the plunger up and down several times. Excess alcohol may cause pain and redness at the site of injection.

4. Read label on insulin bottle to assure use of the correct kind of insulin.

5. Wipe top of bottle with an alcohol swab to sterilize.

Measuring only one type of insulin:

6. Rotate bottle of cloudy insulin in hand (do not shake vigorously, as the resultant bubbles are difficult to remove). As the insulin settles

to the bottom of the bottle it needs to be mixed gently.

7. Draw air into syringe — equal to dose of insulin.

8. Inject air into insulin bottle — to equalize air pressure.

9. Turn the bottle upside-down and draw insulin into syringe. Watch for bubble.

10. Push plunger back into syringe to remove air bubble, and pull back out to correct insulin dose. Be sure to check unit marks.

11. Remove needle from bottle and place on alcohol cotton ball.

Drawing up mixture of long-acting and regular insulin:

6. Rotate bottle of cloudy insulin in hands (as above).

7. Draw air into syringe, equal to the dose of long-acting insulin. Inject air into bottle of long-acting insulin and remove needle without withdrawing insulin.

8. Draw air into syringe, equal to dose of regular insulin. Inject this air into bottle of regular insulin. Turn the bottle upside-down and draw out measured amount of insulin. Watch for and expel bubble, and check unit marks to correct insulin dose.

9. Finally, again insert needle into bottle of long-acting insulin and slowly withdraw the correct amount of this insulin. Do not pull the plunger out too fast, or air bubbles will come into the syringe. If an error is made while drawing up the insulin, the syringe must be emptied and the insulin redrawn.

10. Remove the needle from bottle and place on cotton ball. The insulin is now ready to inject.

SELECTION OF THE INSULIN INJECTION SITE

In selecting the injection spot, certain criteria should be considered:

— Is the site easily accessible? In other words, can the site be used without undue awkwardness in administration?

— Will it allow a smooth, consistent rate of absorption? Certain types of tissue allow a more even rate of absorption than others.

— Is the layer of skin and fat loose enough to be lifted away from the underlying muscle with relative ease?

— Is the site sufficiently lacking in sensitivity? The areas close to the midline of the body, such as the inner aspects of the thighs and arms, are particularly rich in nerve supply. Therefore, injections in these areas are very uncomfortable. The injection of insulin should not be really painful. If it is, it is most probably because of some inaccuracy of technique.

Insulin injection sites are indicated in Fig. 5. Sites accessible for self-injection of insulin are the areas indicated on the thighs and the abdomen. Sites accessible for someone else to inject are the arms and the back. It is better not to use the buttocks unless the layer of fat is loose enough to be easily pinched up and away from the deeper muscle layer.

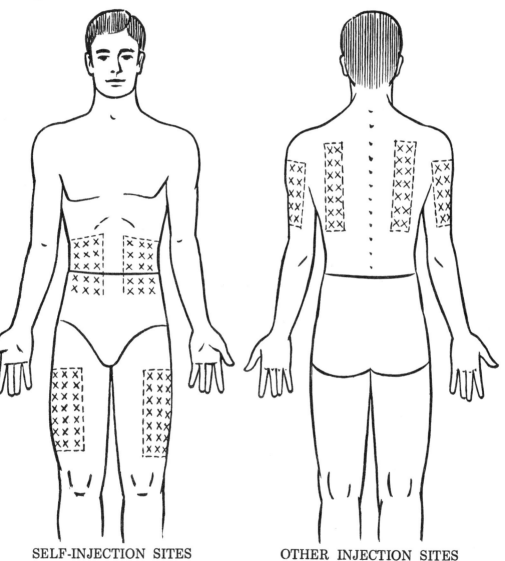

SELF-INJECTION SITES   OTHER INJECTION SITES

FIG. 5 — Suggested sites for Insulin Injection.

It is important to rotate injection areas so that the same site is not used more frequently than every four to six weeks. Repeated injections into the same area leads to thickening of the tissues, resulting in a slower rate of absorption of insulin. Each injection should be approximately 1 to 1½ inches apart to allow complete absorption around the area.

INJECTION OF INSULIN:
- Pinch up the skin with the thumb and forefinger.
- Wipe off skin with an alcohol cotton ball.

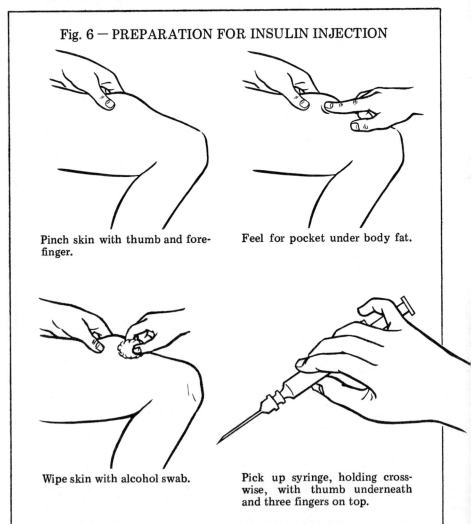

Fig. 6 — PREPARATION FOR INSULIN INJECTION

Pinch skin with thumb and fore-finger.

Feel for pocket under body fat.

Wipe skin with alcohol swab.

Pick up syringe, holding cross-wise, with thumb underneath and three fingers on top.

— Hold syringe crosswise, with thumb on one side and three fingers on the other side (not like a pencil or a dart).

— With the needle parallel to the skin, quickly insert the needle into the skin at the base of the fold. See Fig. 6, 7 and 8.

— Inject the insulin by pressing the plunger in with the little finger.

— Drop the pocket of fat, place the cotton ball over the site of the injection, and withdraw the needle. Do not rub the injection site, but you may hold the cotton ball in place until bleeding, if any, stops.

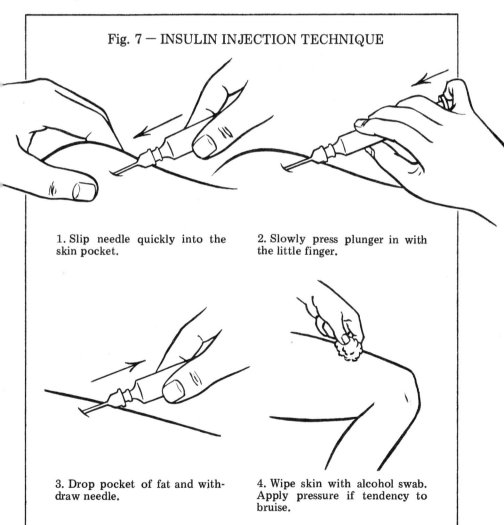

Fig. 7 — INSULIN INJECTION TECHNIQUE

1. Slip needle quickly into the skin pocket.

2. Slowly press plunger in with the little finger.

3. Drop pocket of fat and with-draw needle.

4. Wipe skin with alcohol swab. Apply pressure if tendency to bruise.

LOCAL REACTIONS RESULTING FROM THE INJECTION OF INSULIN

LIPODYSTROPHIES.

Many people who have taken insulin regularly have developed, at the site of injection, one of two fatty tissue responses: fat atrophy, or fat hypertrophy. Fat atrophy appears as depressed, hollow areas at the site of injection due to disappearance of the fatty layer beneath the skin. Hypertrophy, or lumpy, thickened areas at the site of injection, reflect a mild inflammatory reaction in the fatty layer followed by scarring. While no proof of the cause of these tissue changes has been found, or why they occur in some persons and not in others, it is possible that these tissue reactions were due to certain impurities in the insulins used prior to the introduction of the "single peak" insulins (described earlier on p. 86).

The injection technique recommended in this book assumes that repeated injections of other than "single peak" insulins into the same site and/or into the fatty layer may cause these problems.

To decrease the chances for lipodystrophies developing, injection sites should be rotated as described in "Selection of Insulin Site", and

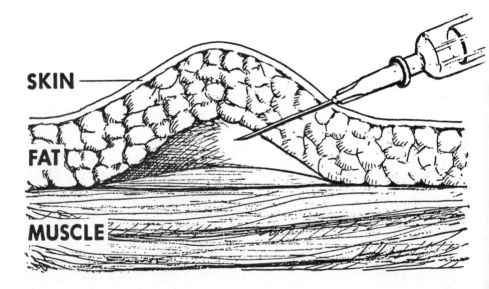

Fig. 8 — Insulin deposited under subcutaneous fat layer; i.e., in subcutaneous space.

needles long enough to reach the area beneath the layer fat should be used. Insulin is absorbed at a more even rate, and there is little irritation when it is injected into this "pocket" area. Obviously, the fat layer is thicker in some people than in others, and even varies from one part of the body to another part. A 5/8 inch needle may be required in one area of the body and a 7/8 inch in another area. To measure for the proper needle length, pick up the skin and fat, and measure the distance across the base of this fold. This distance is the correct needle length.

Where insulin hypertrophy already exists it is best that such areas be allowed to rest and fresh sites be used. These hypertrophic areas may slowly clear, but perhaps not for months. A member of the family should give the injections in the back or arms while the sites recover. In more than 90 percent of persons with lipoatrophy the condition can be successfully resolved by injecting purified "single peak" mixed beef-pork insulins directly into the affected areas. The unsuccessful cases may respond to "single peak" pork insulin or "single component" pork insulin.

INSULIN ALLERGY.

A few people taking insulin for the first time develop raised, tender, reddened areas at the site of each insulin injection. Each allergic response persists up to 24 hours. If this should occur, consult your physician. However, the following points might be considered:

— Be sure that excess alcohol is removed from the syringe and needle, and that the cotton ball is squeezed out before wiping the skin. This may occasionally be a factor. Some people who are especially sensitive to alcohol would do better to boil their syringe each day rather than keep it in alcohol.

— If insulins other than purified "single peak" are being used, consult with your physician about changing to them. If the local skin allergy persists, then arrangements can be made to try "single component" beef or pork insulin.

— Be sure you are injecting deep enough with a long enough needle. Superficial injections are often the cause of these types of areas.

BRUISES AT THE SITE OF INSULIN INJECTION.

These may appear in individuals with heavy thighs and, in particular, if many small veins are visible in the skin of the thighs. This does not prevent the use of these areas for insulin injection. The bruises can be controlled by immediately applying pressure to the injection point for twenty or thirty seconds following removal of the needle.

ADJUSTMENT OF INSULIN DOSE

The level of blood glucose can fluctuate widely in the insulin-dependent diabetic. This is not unusual and is only of real significance if (1) it is associated with frequent attacks of hypoglycemia; (2) it leads to prolonged periods of poorly-controlled diabetes. An appreciation of the reasons for hypoglycemia or for persistent elevations of blood glucose levels can assist in better home management of D.M.

Within the cyclic patterns of daily living things happen which lead to **elevated blood glucose values** such as: (1) dietary excesses, particularly of carbohydrate foods; (2) inactivity; (3) emotional and other stresses; (4) insufficient insulin action. These influences are frequently the cause of sporadic 0.5 to 2 percent glucose in the urine. This is not serious. However, if the urine tests begin to regularly show in excess of one percent this may lead to uncontrolled diabetes. Since it is important to prevent uncontrolled diabetes, **corrective measures** should be considered. First, consider the causes of an elevated blood glucose. If it is a dietary indiscretion, return for a time to the use of a measured diet. If there are no symptoms of an infection the second step is to consider an adjustment of the insulin dose. In the event of an infection associated with a fever, follow the recommendations on page 116.

☐ *FACTORS WHICH RAISE BLOOD SUGAR*

Increase in food intake
   (particularly carbohydrate)
Decrease in physical activity
Stress:
   Infection
   Severe injury or surgery
   Emotional strain
   Pregnancy
Impaired insulin absorption
   (faulty technique)

If hypoglycemic reactions are occurring with some frequency, i.e. more than two mild ones per week or any severe reaction, again it is well to consider the reasons for their occurrence and, if the reason is not obvious, plan an adjustment of the insulin dose. The obvious reasons are generally excessive or unusual exercise, being late for a meal, or too little food. If there is no apparent cause for hypoglycemia then the insulin dose should be decreased.

□ *FACTORS WHICH LOWER BLOOD SUGAR*

Decrease in food intake.
Delay in meal hour.
Increase in physical activity.
Recovery from stress.
Decrease in insulin requirement.
> e.g. Milder diabetes —
>> Improved absorption due to
>> change in injection technique.

GUIDELINES FOR ADJUSTMENT OF INSULIN DOSE — WITH THE CONSENT OF YOUR PHYSICIAN.

General Considerations:

1. No adjustment is made in dose when spilling glucose in urine or when hypoglycemic reactions are the result of a **temporary** upset in the daily routine.

2. If the urine test for glucose is persistently one percent or higher throughout the day, or at one time of the day for a three day period,
   A. **Increase** the insulin **2 units** if the total daily dose is 30 units or less.
   B. **Increase** the insulin **4 units** if the total daily dose is more than 30 units.

3. If hypoglycemia occurs as a mild reaction **twice in one week** or as a more severe reaction on one occasion without apparent reason, decrease the insulin **2 units** (for a mild reaction) or **4 units** (for a severe reaction. A large decrease may be in order when the daily insulin dose is more) than 30 or 40 units daily.

4. These are only general guidelines and may need individual modification by your doctor.

ADJUSTMENT OF A SINGLE DAILY INSULIN DOSE

THE DOSE IS INCREASED IF	*Insulin to Increase*
Glucose is present in urine over a 3 day period.	
— Before breakfast each day	— Increase NPH or Lente
— Before lunch	— Increase Regular
— Before lunch and supper each day	— Increase Regular
— Uncertain what to do	— Consult physician

INSULIN ACTION CURVES

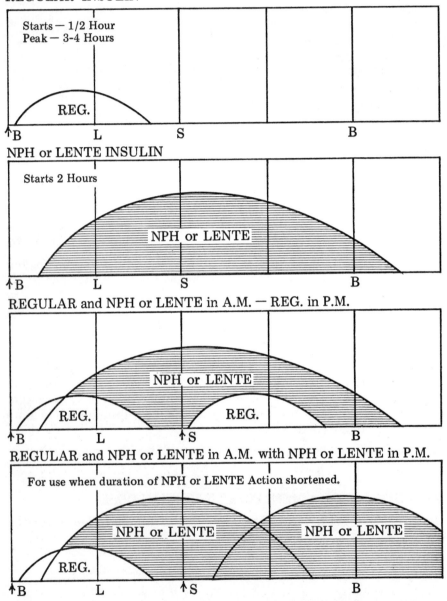

REGULAR INSULIN

Starts — 1/2 Hour
Peak — 3-4 Hours

REG.

B   L   S   B

NPH or LENTE INSULIN

Starts 2 Hours

NPH or LENTE

B   L   S   B

REGULAR and NPH or LENTE in A.M. — REG. in P.M.

NPH or LENTE

REG.   REG.

B   L   S   B

REGULAR and NPH or LENTE in A.M. with NPH or LENTE in P.M.

For use when duration of NPH or LENTE Action shortened.

NPH or LENTE   NPH or LENTE

REG.

B   L   S   B

Fig. 9
↑point or time of insulin injection B-L-S—mealtimes

THE DOSE IS DECREASED IF	*Insulin to Decrease*
Hypoglycemic reactions are occurring two or more times a week.	
— For reactions occurring before lunch or before supper	— Decrease Regular
— For reactions occurring sometime after supper, i.e. during the night or before breakfast.	— Decrease NPH or Lente.

ADJUSTMENT OF A SPLIT DAILY INSULIN DOSE

THE DOSE IS INCREASED IF	*Insulin to Increase*
Glucose is present in urine over a 3 day period.	
— Before breakfast each day	— Increase evening NPH or Lente
— Before lunch each day	— Increase morning Regular
— Before breakfast and lunch	— Increase evening NPH or Lente
— Before supper each day	— Increase morning NPH or Lente
— At bedtime daily	— Increase evening Regular

THE DOSE IS DECREASED IF	*Insulin to Decrease*
Hypoglicemic reactions are occurring two or more times a week.	
— For reactions before lunch	— Decrease morning Regular
— For reactions late in afternoon	— Decrease morning NPH or Lente
— For reactions in early evening	— Decrease evening Regular
— For reactions in early hours before breakfast	— Decrease evening NPH or Lente

The reasons for the above recommendations relate to the time action curves of insulin action as demonstrated for the various kinds of insulin in Fig. 9.

CARE OF INSULIN WHILE TRAVELING

When traveling it is advisable to keep your insulin and other equipment close at hand. Insulin will need to be protected from excessive temperatures, such as the low temperatures in the baggage sections of some aircraft and the heat during summer travel. Although many types of carrying containers have been manufactured for the convenience of insulin-dependent patients, they often are expensive and bulky to carry. An inexpensive wide-mouth thermos with a freezer lid will hold at least four bottles of insulin. If the lid is kept in the refrigerator freezer prior to traveling, when placed on the thermos it will keep the insulin cool for several hours. The insulation of the container itself should keep insulin at about room temperature. The new purified insulins are stable at room temperature for at least a year. Disposable syringes and needles and packaged alcohol wipes make taking insulin away from home much easier. Additional travel suggestions are given in Part V, Chapter 16.

[1] Albisser, A. M., et al, (1974) Clinical Control of Diabetes by the Artificial Pancreas. *Diabetes* 23:397.

[2] Soeldner, J. S. et al, (1973) In Vitro and In Vivo Experience with a Miniature Glucose Sensor. *Diabetes* 22:(Suppl. 1) 294.

[3] Lazarow, A. et al, (1973) Islet Differentiation, Organ Culture, and Transplantation. *Diabetes* 22:877.

[4] Amamoo, D. G., et al, (1974) Preliminary Experience with Pancreatic Islet — Cell Implantation. *Mayo Clinic Proceedings* 49:289.

[5] Special Report (1974) Position Paper on Pancreatic Islet and Beta Cell Transplantation in Man. *Diabetes* 23:987.

Chapter 8   HYPOGLYCEMIA

NATURE OF HYPOGLYCEMIA

Hypoglycemia means a low level of blood glucose, usually below 60 mg. The physical effect of a low blood sugar commonly is called an "insulin reaction," since it is usually experienced by persons administering insulin. However, as there are a number of reasons for an abnormally low blood glucose, the designation "insulin reaction" is misleading.* Persons receiving such oral treatment as Orinase, Diabinese, Dymelor or Tolinase can develop a low blood glucose level. It is therefore much better to use the term HYPOGLYCEMIA. Symptoms characteristic of hypoglycemia are more likely to occur with blood glucose values less than 50 mg. (plasma value below 60 mg.).

*Hypoglycemia occasionally occurs in some very mild diabetics who are overweight and in some non-diabetics who are nervous and tense, or have an organic disease leading to over-production of insulin.

Though there are times when hypoglycemia fails to produce any noticeable effects, at least mild symptoms often result. For some, the attacks may be distressing and on occasion may be temporarily incapacitating. It is therefore necessary to understand the nature of hypoglycemia and its prevention.

The symptoms of hypoglycemia vary from person to person. This is due in part to the function of the sympathetic nerves — nerves that cause a blush during embarrassment or heart palpitations with fright. A drop in blood glucose causes these nerves to bring about the release of a substance from the adrenal gland known as epinephrine. Epinephrine produces rather specific symptoms. If the nerves are not healthy and functioning well, epinephrine may not be effectively released and the blood glucose level may continue to fall. This can lead to an interference in the function of the cerebral cortex (brain cells) causing a different set of symptoms from hypoglycemia.

The release of epinephrine serves two very useful functions. It causes early warning signals of hypoglycemia and it helps to correct the low level of blood glucose.

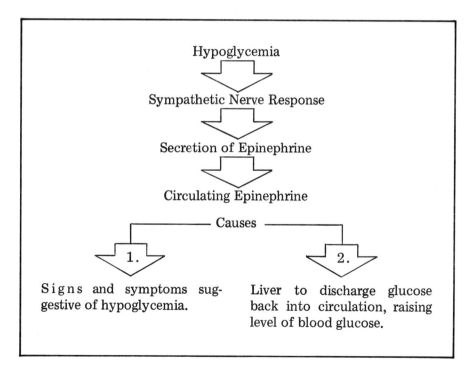

TYPES OF HYPOGLYCEMIA REACTIONS AND THE RESULTING SIGNS AND SYMPTOMS

EPINEPHRINE can be responsible for such warning signs as:
Hunger
A nervous, shaky feeling
Irritability
Sweating
Palpitations of the heart
Tingling and numbness of the lips and tongue

CEREBRAL CORTEX EFFECT

The cerebral brain cells cannot function well if deprived of oxygen or glucose. This is demonstrated by one or more of the signs listed below. There is frequently an inability to recognize what is happening resulting in delay or failure to start corrective measures.

Such complaints as those listed below may be the result of hypoglycemia.
Headache
Faintness
Blurred vision
Difficulty with making decisions, mental confusion

Evidences of hypoglycemia may include:
Weakness
Tremor
Staggering gait
Behavioral changes
Loss of consciousness

The signs and symptoms of hypoglycemia usually occur some hours (more than three or four) after eating. If similar symptoms occur within two hours of having eaten, other causes for the symptoms should be considered, such as anxiety or nervous tension, which can also cause an epinephrine effect. Infrequently hypoglycemia may be present at the start of the meal causing a delay in the digestion and absorption of food eaten at the meal. The hypoglycemic state may then persist past the meal hour. When the symptoms are experienced before an approaching meal, they should be considered due to hypoglycemia and treated accordingly. If there is uncertainty about the cause of the symptoms, follow the recommendations for the treatment of hypoglycemia and discuss the problem later with your physician.

CAUSES AND PREVENTION OF HYPOGLYCEMIA

Prevention depends first on recognizing and then correcting those practices which lead to hypoglycemia. Prevention also depends upon the acceptance of some rigidity of a daily routine. It is important to arise and take insulin at nearly the same hour each day. Regularity of eating hours and constancy of food intake are necessary. Daily exercise is beneficial, but it requires certain precautions when carried out in an excessive or irregular manner. Alcohol cannot be used in excess, since it can either mask the symptoms of hypoglycemia or, on the other hand, produce symptoms suggestive of hypoglycemia. Its use can interfere with the keeping of regular meal hours and, additionally, alcohol in the absence of food can promote hypoglycemia.

Exercise is encouraged for all, particularly the young with diabetes. Young people should not be discouraged from participating in track, tennis, volleyball, football, basketball, hockey, golf, hiking or mountain climbing or other physical activities. However, it is important to prepare for these activities by eating sufficiently, having an adjustment of insulin dosage, and taking supplementary sweets during some of these activities. Reportedly, the well known former Notre Dame quarterback, Coley O'Brien, who was discovered to have diabetes in his adolescence, required a daily intake of 5,000 calories during the football season. Bill Talbert, the famous Davis Cup tennis star and coach who developed juvenile diabetes, reportedly sipped Coca-Cola during his tennis matches to provide energy and to prevent hypoglycemia. Some people planning a morning round of golf reduce their morning insulin dose (usually the regular insulin) by some 6 to 8 units.

If there is difficulty recognizing hypoglycemia, it is advisable to arrange for a family member, fellow worker or school teacher to look for signs of hypoglycemia and assist in carrying out the appropriate treatment. Furthermore, it is often advantageous (particularly for children) to have between-meal and bedtime feedings.

☐ ALWAYS CARRY DIABETIC IDENTIFICATION

There is one other precaution. Sometimes the epinephrine effect after hypoglycemia causes the following urine test for glucose to be strongly positive. If this is followed by an increase in insulin dose, further low blood glucose levels will occur. This variable pattern of control; i.e., Somogyi Effect, will only improve when the dose of insulin is first decreased so as to prevent hypoglycemia.

TREATMENT OF HYPOGLYCEMIA

WHEN TO TREAT

1. If you think you are having hypoglycemia — treat.

2. If you are not sure whether or not you having hypoglycemia, again, treat — then consider the problem.

If the symptoms occurred two or more hours after a meal, hypoglycemia is a possibility. However, if the symptoms came shortly after a meal, hypoglycemia is less likely.

3. If hypoglycemia occurs within a few minutes of an approaching meal, treat the reaction. After the symptoms have improved, eat the meal. At times hypoglycemia is associated with a spasm of the stomach outlet. If solid food is taken nausea may result, and this may interfere with further oral treatment.

4. If the treatment of hypoglycemia occurs more than an hour before the next meal, additional food should be ingested after recovery, e.g. a glass of milk if there is an hour or two before the next meal, or half a meat sandwich and a glass of milk if the reaction occurs in the late evening or early morning hours.

SUGGESTED TREATMENT

1. Epinephrine effect: mild, i.e. symptoms are felt but no signs are evident.

    1/2 glass of orange or other fruit juice, 7-Up, ginger ale, Pepsi or Coke.

2. Epinephrine effect: moderate, i.e. symptoms are felt and sweating and tremulousness are present.
    A. Add 1 tsp. of sugar to 1/2 glass of fruit juice, or take a full glass of carbonated beverage.
    B. 4-5 cubes of sugar (not 1 or 2 lifesavers — not a chocolate bar. The two lifesavers are not enough sugar. The chocolate bar may be difficult for some to swallow).

3. Cerebral effect: severe manifestations are present. A family member, colleague, friend previously informed will have to direct treatment.
    A. If there is no difficulty swallowing, give 1 tsp. of sugar in 1/4 glass of orange juice and repeat in a few minutes. On recovery give a glass of milk or feeding of similar food value.
    B. If unable to swallow, have available for use at home:
       1) Glucagon (by prescription only)

(3-B-1, Cont.)
    a. Give a child 1/2 mg. subcutaneously.
    b. Give an adult 1 mg. subcutaneously.
    Give in the same manner insulin is injected.

Glucagon, like insulin, is produced in the pancreas. It is a secretion of the alpha cell of the Islets of Langerhans and is capable of raising the blood glucose level by causing the release of stored glucose from the liver.

Glucagon is best used for the treatment of a hypoglycemic reaction accompanied by drowsiness, inability to swallow, or nausea. It should be injected subcutaneously as one injects insulin, using the same equipment. Half a vial is used in a child and a full dose (1 mg.) is used in the adult. If improvement is not seen in twenty minutes, the injection may be repeated. One should be familiar with the directions for preparing glucagon for injection (see brochure with package), as well as with the technique of giving the injection.

If the person is unconscious, then place face down to prevent choking if vomiting occurs. After responding to glucagon and/or instant glucose, give a sweetened drink followed by a more substantial feeding, such as a glass of milk, half a cheese or peanut butter sandwich, etc.

The following recommendations regarding the use of glucagon are made:
1. The ampule should be kept in storage under refrigeration.
2. The technique of preparation and administration are clearly outlined in the brochure accompanying the medication. Members of the family should be familiar with this before the emergency arises. The actual injection is made in the same manner as with insulin.
3. Glucagon should be given promptly when it is apparent that the patient cannot or will not take sugar.
4. After awakening, the patient should promptly take sugar in the form of fruit juice, carbonated beverage, etc. If the reaction occurs more than an hour before another meal, food containing protein should be taken, e.g. 200 grams (a full glass) of milk or half of a meat or cheese sandwich.

  5. The physician should be called promptly. If the patient
     has not improved within 15 minutes, it may be neces-
     sary to administer glucose intravenously.
2) Instant Glucose (available through the Cleveland Diabetes
   Association).*
   Small amounts are repeatedly placed inside the cheek from
   where it can be absorbed.

   Instant glucose is a concentrated form of glucose in a jelly-like
   consistency which comes in a tube. Administer by squirting
   the material inside the cheek and massaging the glucose directly into the blood stream from the mucous membrane,
   thus raising the blood sugar level. Give about 1/5 to 1/4 of the
   tube at a time. Repeat the administration every few minutes
   until the full amount has been given. If the patient is not
   arousing, follow other measures as previously outlined.

Fig. 10 is a summary of the causes, signs and symptoms and treatment
of hypoglycemia.

HYPOGLYCEMIA AND DRIVERS LICENSES

In many states a drivers license may be suspended for loss of consciousness or loss of ability to drive properly due to hypoglycemia. For this
reason, many diabetics should eat 10 or 15 grams of carbohydrate
(medium sized orange, apple, or two to three graham crackers) before
driving home from work. Always have graham crackers, chocolate or
sugar cubes in the glove compartment of your car, in the desk or locker
at work, or in your purse. Such aids are not only valuable for the
treatment of hypoglycemia, but can be taken to ward off hypoglycemia
if a regular meal is delayed.

*Refer to Resource List, p. 182.

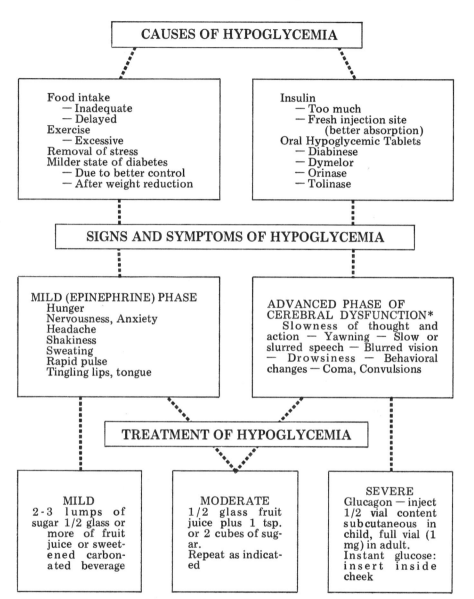

CAUSES OF HYPOGLYCEMIA

Food intake
  — Inadequate
  — Delayed
Exercise
  — Excessive
Removal of stress
Milder state of diabetes
  — Due to better control
  — After weight reduction

Insulin
  — Too much
  — Fresh injection site
    (better absorption)
Oral Hypoglycemic Tablets
  — Diabinese
  — Dymelor
  — Orinase
  — Tolinase

SIGNS AND SYMPTOMS OF HYPOGLYCEMIA

MILD (EPINEPHRINE) PHASE
  Hunger
  Nervousness, Anxiety
  Headache
  Shakiness
  Sweating
  Rapid pulse
  Tingling lips, tongue

ADVANCED PHASE OF
CEREBRAL DYSFUNCTION*
  Slowness of thought and
  action — Yawning — Slow or
  slurred speech — Blurred vision
  — Drowsiness — Behavioral
  changes — Coma, Convulsions

TREATMENT OF HYPOGLYCEMIA

MILD
2-3 lumps of
sugar 1/2 glass or
more of fruit
juice or sweet-
ened carbon-
ated beverage

MODERATE
1/2 glass fruit
juice plus 1 tsp.
or 2 cubes of sug-
ar.
Repeat as indicat-
ed

SEVERE
Glucagon — inject
1/2 vial content
subcutaneous in
child, full vial (1
mg) in adult.
Instant glucose:
insert inside
cheek

FIG. 10 — Summary of causes, signs and symptoms, and treatment of Hypo-glycemia in D.M.

*People with a past history of having had difficulty with the recognition of hypo-glycemia should always have someone nearby; e.g., a family member at home or on outings, a teacher, a fellow worker, or colleague who is familiar with the problem; i.e., how to recognize the signs of impending hypoglycemia, where to locate and how to administer the sugar or other materials for the treatment of hypoglycemia.

Chapter 9 URINE TESTS FOR SUGAR AND KETONES

REASONS TO TEST THE URINE

A number of tests can be used to check for the presence of sugar and ketones in the urine. The tests are performed on a regular basis, at the suggestion of the physician, to provide information about the degree of control of diabetes. We know that blood glucose levels in excess of the kidney's capacity to reabsorb sugar (the "spilling point" for glucose) leads to loss of glucose from the body. In small amounts loss of glucose in the urine may be of little importance. However, large amounts may lead to symptoms of uncontrolled diabetes. Regular testing of the urine for glucose is valuable for this reason. A changing pattern of test results will call attention to the need to re-evaluate one's diabetic management routine. In this way conditions leading to loss of control of diabetes may be corrected (See page 96).

Tests for glucose and ketones are an inexpensive and simple way of assisting in the home care of diabetes. A record book of test results should be presented to the physician during regular office visits.

TESTS FOR GLUCOSE IN THE URINE

Considerations for a specific test are: simplicity, ease of interpretation, and cost. The latter factor may be of little importance for those performing only one test a day.

The test materials most often used are:
1. Clinitest Tablets (Ames Company).
These tablets of a copper salt were developed after many years use of the Benedicts solution of the copper salt. They are a very satisfactory and inexpensive means of testing the urine for glucose. This test may not be quite as sensitive as the more expensive paper or strip tests.

2. Paper or plastic strip tests are very specific for glucose. This is because the test material contains a substance (enzyme) called glucose oxidase. Examples are:
   Clinistix (Ames Company)
   Tes-Tape (Lilly Company)
   Diastix (Ames Company)

On the basis of cost and ease of interpretation Clinitest tablets might serve best for those testing their urine more than once a day. Diastix is also quite useful but is more costly. For adults not using insulin who test less frequently and are less likely to show more than small amounts of glucose, the paper strip tests may be quite useful. The latter tests are certainly simpler to use away from home. Where there are small children in the home it might be safer to use the paper or plastic stip test. Consult with your doctor about his preference.

Accuracy in performing the test is most important. Read the directions accompanying the various tests thoroughly before using them. Be sure to time the tests carefully as directed.

*TESTS AND TEST MATERIALS**

1. Clinitest — two methods
   Materials needed:

Clinitest tablets	Color chart
Clean test tube	Clean water
(comes in Clinitest kit)	Urine collection container
Eye dropper	Urine test record

   A. 5 drop method:
      1) Put 10 drops of water into test tube.
      2) Put 5 drops of urine into test tube.
      3) Add 1 Clinitest tablet. The tablet will cause the urine and water to bubble up.
      4) After the bubbling has stopped, count slowly to 15, or measure **15 seconds** on the sweep second hand of a watch.
      5) Gently shake the test tube and then compare immediately with the Clinitest color chart.
      6) Record the results in the urine test record (as shown below):

0 for Negative	1/2% for 1+	1% for 3+
1/4% for Trace	3/4% for 2+	2% for 4+

      Recording in terms of percent rather than pluses is a more accurate interpretation of test results.
      7) Keep Clinitest bottle tightly capped and in a dry, cool place. Clinitest tablets deteriorate if exposed to moisture and light, resulting in falsely negative tests. Be certain to

*Film strips on urine testing are available. See resource materials, page 182.

read and follow carefully the manufacturer's instructions regarding care and inspection of tablets. Do not use tablets which have turned blue in color.

B. 2 drop method:

Any time the test turns bright orange during the bubbling period and then becomes a dark brown or muddy color after counting to 15, it means that there is actually more than 2% sugar in the specimen. The tests can then be repeated using the 2 drop method which will register up to 5% sugar. A special 2-drop color chart is necessary for comparison.

1) Put 10 drops of water into test tube.
2) Put 2 drops of urine into test tube.
3) Add 1 Clinitest tablet.
4) After the bubbling has stopped, count slowly to 15.
5) Gently shake the test tube and compare with the 2 drop Clinitest color chart.
6) Record results in urine test record according to the color chart in the kit.

0 for Negative	½%	2%
Trace	1%	3%
		5%

☐ *TO INSURE ACCURACY OF TEST*

Dip
Time Test
Compare with color chart

2. **Diastix**
Follow the directions on the package insert.

3. **Tes-Tape**
Follow the directions on the package insert.

4. **Clinistix**
Follow the directions on the package insert. Use percentages to record the results.

DRUGS WHICH MAY AFFECT RESULTS OF URINE TESTS FOR GLUCOSE

1. Clinitest: the result may appear as a false positive when the following medicines are being used:
   A. Antibiotics, e.g. penicillin, Keflex, Neg-gram.
   B. INH for tuberculosis

C. Aspirin
D. Vitamin C
E. Benemid
F. L-Dopa
G. Chloral Hydrate

2. Enzyme paper or strip test: may show negative even in the presence of glucose when the urine specimen is collected from persons taking:
   A. Vitamin C (large dose intake)
   B. L-Dopa
   C. Methyl Dopa

TIME OF URINE COLLECTION FOR GLUCOSE TEST

Different times to test the urine are suggested, depending upon which treatment plan is being followed.

Treatment Plan	When to Test
Diet alone Diet and diabetic pill	Test urine specimen passed 1½ hours after breakfast or other meal. This does not have to be a second-voiding. See page 10.
Diet and insulin	1. Empty bladder about an hour **before** meals, drink a glass of water, and in 30-40 minutes pass urine again and test. These second-voided specimens are to be done daily **before** breakfast and **before** supper, and **before** lunch and at bedtime if so directed. 2. Your physician may wish a test of the first voided specimen in the morning to evaluate night time control.

24 HOUR URINE COLLECTION

Single urine specimens and blood glucose tests tell only what the control is at the moment the specimen is collected. Therefore, it is of value to periodically test a sample of a 24 hour urine collection, which gives some indication of the degree of control for the whole day. A specimen at the time of a visit to your physician can be tested "quantitatively" and, knowing the total volume, the actual number of grams of sugar spilled over the 24 hour period can be calculated.

Materials needed:

Large clean, empty container: cider jug, plastic gallon container.
Benzoic Acid Crystals or 2.5 Gm. tablets
Boric acid crystals or 2.5 Gm. tablets
Measuring cup and spoons
Small specimen bottle
Put 1 tablet or 1 tablespoon boric acid or benzoic acid crystals in the bottom of the clean, empty gallon jug prior to the collection. These materials act as a preservative to help prevent odor during the period of collection, and also act to keep bacteria from multiplying in the specimen.

Method of collection:

The day before a visit to the doctor save all the urine passed in 24 hours.

1. Empty bladder before breakfast on the first day of the collection and discard this urine.

2. Save all urine collected for the rest of the day, including the first voided specimen the next morning (this will be a full 24 hours).

3. Fill a small specimen bottle with the sample of collected urine and label the bottle with your name, date collected.

4. Measure the total amount of urine and record it in cups or ounces.

5. Write the total volume of urine on the specimen label. Take this sample with you to the physician's office.

TESTS FOR ACETONE (KETONES OR KETONE BODIES) IN THE URINE

A possibility exists for developing ketoacidosis whenever the urine tests, particularly in the presence of an acute illness, indicate uncontrolled diabetes. When this happens acetone is passed in the urine and can be detected by appropriate testing. This test should be performed whenever urine tests show 2 percent or more for glucose.

The tests to use:

Acetest tablets (Ames Co.)

Follow the directions on the bottle. Record the results in the urine test record.

Ketostix (Ames Co.)

1. Dip Ketostix into urine specimen and remove.
2. Count 15 seconds.
3. Compare immediately with the Ketostix color chart.
4. Record results in the urine test record.
   O for Negative   Moderate*
   Small   Large*

Ketodiastix (Ames Co.)

The Ketodiastix is a combination stick which might be quite useful for those individuals who are showing increasing amounts of glucose in the urine. This makes it possible to test for glucose and ketones at the same time. Obviously, care must be taken to read the two color tabs at the proper time. These sticks are somewhat more expensive to use, and certainly would not be necessary when the urine glucose is less than 2 percent. Be sure to follow the directions on the package.

KEEPING RECORDS OF URINE TESTS

Simple but carefully and consistently kept records can be of great value to the patient and physician in managing diabetes, when the records for a few weeks or months are available for review. Patterns in spilling of glucose or hypoglycemia may assist in recognizing the cause or causes for the fluctuations in control and help to initiate appropriate measures for their correction. These records need not be complicated, and will probably take about 1/2 minute a day to keep.

What should appear in the records:

1. Results and time of single specimen.

2. Results of tests for acetone (whenever urine test for sugar shows 2 percent or more).

3. Insulin dose and type of insulin used.

4. Hypoglycemic reactions — degree and time of day.

5. Diet and weekly weight.

6. Any unusual circumstances which might explain unusual spilling of sugar or the occurrence of low blood sugar reactions.

*If you do not feel well and urine test for acetone shows moderate or large amount, contact your physician.

Forms for records

When records are to be mailed in, printed slips of suitable size may be used. When the report is presented to the physician, a small, pocket size spiral type notebook is considerably more convenient. The information should be arranged somewhat as follows:

TWO WEEKS BEGINNING _____						BODY WEIGHT _____ C _____ P_____ F_____					
DATE	URINE SUGAR				KETONES	INSULIN OR ORAL TABLET		INSULIN REACTION		REMARKS
	A. M.	N.	P. M.	BED		A. M.	P. M.	A. M.	P. M.	
SUN										
MON										
TUES										
WED										
THURS										
FRI										
SAT										
SUN										
MON										
TUES										
WED										
THURS										
FRI										
SAT										

Chapter 10 ACUTE ILLNESS ROUTINES FOR MANAGEMENT OF DM

Whenever an acute illness strikes, particularly one that is accompanied by fever or pain, or which interferes with dietary intake, it is helpful to have a program ready to follow.

STOMACH FLU (GASTROENTERITIS)

The problem with gastroenteritis is one of nausea, abdominal cramps, and diarrhea, which prevent the use of a general diabetic diet. If vomiting occurs, oral intake is usually not possible.

It will be helpful to:

1. Test the urine for glucose. If over 1 percent, test for ketones.

2. Check oral temperature.

3. Contact the physician. He will want to know about the urine test for glucose and ketones and whether there is any fever. He may wish to prescribe medication for nausea or diarrhea, if troublesome.

4. If there is freedom from fever and inability to take a full liquid diet:
   1) Test the urine for glucose and if the result is **1 percent or less** on rising in the morning:
      — Take 1/2 of the usual a.m. insulin dose.
      — Drink by sips approximately 1/2 glass (120 grams) of 7-Up, ginger ale or apple juice each hour over a 10 to 12 hour period.
      — Later in the day, at noon and at 6 p.m., if the urine test for glucose shows 1 percent, take an additional amount of regular insulin equal to 1/4 of the total a.m. dose. If the test result is 2 percent, take the remaining 1/2 of the a.m. dose instead.
   2) If the urine test for glucose is **2 percent or more** on the morning of the illness, it will be best to take the full dose of insulin. If **ketones** are present in addition, the patient should contact his physician as he may wish to prescribe additional amounts of insulin.
      — Continue to test the urine every 4 to 6 hours for glucose and ketones. If there is difficulty with the control of diabetes, report this to the physician or the nurse clinician.
      — Take fluids hourly as directed above, with the addition of a cup of broth every 3 hours. If the patient cannot take fluids by mouth or if vomiting ensues, the physician may wish to

arrange intravenous administration of fluids.

3) For those with milder diabetes and not taking insulin:
   — Test the urine for glucose once or twice daily. If the urine begins to show over 1 percent glucose, notify the physician.
   — If oral diabetic pills are usually taken, they may be omitted for a few hours. The blood level of the medicine persists for six or more hours. Their use may be resumed later when vomiting is controlled.

ACUTE ILLNESS WITH FEVER

Many acute illnesses causing temperatures of 100 degrees or more are managed at home, e.g., influenza, acute bronchitis, Strep. throat, measles and mumps. These illnesses are associated with a stress response which leads to insufficient action of insulin in the diabetic. This in turn leads to an increase in insulin requirement. In addition, as one's sense of well-being is adversely affected there is a loss of appetite and lessening of physical activity. At such times it is well to have a plan to follow. One such plan:

1. Test the urine for glucose. If the test shows glucose in excess of 1 percent (or 3+), also test for ketones. Repeat the test every 4 to 6 hours. This information is important to the physician.

2. Contact the physician.

3. Have a liquid diet to use. Example diets follow. A liquid feeding every three hours, five feedings a day, can be used if one is suffering from nausea or loss of appetite.

4. Take the usual morning dose of insulin. Supplementary amounts of regular insulin are beneficial before lunch, dinner and even at bedtime when the urine test indicates increasing amounts of glucose. The dose of insulin should be that suggested by a physician. An example of how much regular insulin might be administered based on the result of the urine test for glucose and ketones at the times noted while feverish, is shown in Fig. 11. This is a routine that could be used by an adolescent or adult taking a total of 20 to 60 units of insulin daily.

HOUSEHOLD MEASURE LIQUID DIETS

This diet is for use when ill and poor appetite or nausea make the usual diet impractical.

Eat five times a day at three hour intervals. Each grouping equals one meal. A meat exchange in the form of an egg may be added to any meal.

UNITS OF REGULAR (CZI) INSULIN RECOMMENDED BY URINE TEST DURING ILLNESS WITH FEVER WITH KETONES			
URINE GLUCOSE	ZERO	MODERATE	LARGE
	Insulin units		
0	0		
tr.	0		
1/2%	0		
3/4%	4- 6		
1%	6- 8	8-10	12-14
2%	8-10	10-12	14-16

FIG. 11 — Suggested plan for injecting extra units regular insulin before meals, during illness with fever, based on urine test results for glucose and ketones.

During illness these foods may also be useful:

    7-Up or Ginger Ale - 1/2 cup = 1 fruit exchange

    Meritene - 3 tbsp. = 1 milk exchange

    Metrecal - 1 cup = 1 milk exchange

LIQUID DIET #1

Total Value — C-120; P-60; F-45 gm.

Per Feeding — C-24; P-12, F-9 gm.

1. 3 tbsp. Meritene
   1 cup milk

2. 1/2 cup Cream of Wheat or Cream of Rice
   1/2 cup milk
   1/2 slice toast

3. 1 slice toast
   1/2 cup milk **or** 1/2 cup fruit juice

4. 1 cup soup (diluted)
   7 saltines **or** 1 slice toast

5. 1 cup milk
   1/2 cup fruit juice i.e., orange, apple juice

(Liquid Diet #1 Cont.)

6. 1 cup soup (diluted)
   1/2 cup milk
   3 saltines **or** 1/2 slice toast

7. 1/2 cup ice cream
   1/2 slice toast **or** 3 saltines

8. Metrecal — 1 cup

9. 1/2 cup Jello
   1/2 slice toast **or** 3 saltines

10. 1-1/2 slices toast **or** 9 saltines

11. 1/2 cup 7-Up **or** Ginger Ale

NOTE: Broth or bouillon may be taken as desired.

LIQUID DIET #2
Total Value C-130; P-60; F-60 gm.
Per Feeding C-26; P-12; F-12 gm.

1. 4 tbsp. Meritene
   1 cup milk

2. 1/2 cup Cream of Wheat or Cream of Rice
   1/2 cup milk
   1/2 slice toast

3. 1 slice toast + 1 cup milk **or** 1 fruit

4. 1 cup soup (diluted)
   7 saltines **or** 1 slice toast

5. 1/2 cup 7-Up + 7 saltines **or** 1 slice toast

6. 1 cup soup (diluted)
   1/2 cup milk
   4 saltines **or** 1/2 slice bread

7. Scant 1/2 cup ice cream
   1 slice toast **or** 7 saltines

8. 1/2 cup Metrecal
   1 fruit i.e. half-cup orange, apple or pineapple juice

9. 1/2 cup Jello
   1/2 slice toast **or** 3 saltines

10. 1 fruit (see #8)
    1 slice toast **or** 7 saltines

11. 1/2 cup 7-Up **or** Ginger Ale

NOTE: Broth or bouillon may be taken as desired.

LIQUID DIET #3
Total Value C=150; P-75; F-60 gm.
Per Feeding C-30; P-15; F-12 gm.

1. 4 tbsp. Meritene
   1 cup milk
   1/2 slice toast

2. 1 slice bread or 3 graham crackers
   1 cup milk

3. 1/2 cup milk
   3/4 cup cooked cereal

4. 1 fruit i.e. half-cup orange, apple, or pineapple juice
   1/2 cup milk
   1 slice bread or 3 graham crackers

5. 1-1/2 fruit i.e. three-quarters cup of juice — see #4
   1 slice bread or 7 saltines

6. 1/3 cup Jello
   7 saltines
   1 cup soup (diluted)

7. 1 cup soup (diluted)
   1-1/2 slices bread or 10 saltines

8. 1/2 cup ice cream
   1 slice toast or 7 saltines

9. 1/2 cup Metrecal
   1 slice toast or 3 graham crackers   NOTE: Broth or bouillon may

10. 1 cup 7-Up or Ginger Ale   be taken as desired.

LIQUID DIET #4
Total Value C=180; P=80; F=80 gm.
Per Feeding C-36; P-16; F-16 gm.

1. 4 tbsp. Meritene
   1 cup milk
   1/2 slice toast

2. 1-1/2 slices bread or 3 graham crackers or 7 saltines
   1 cup milk

3. 1/2 cup milk
   1 cup cooked cereal

4. 1 fruit i.e. half-cup orange, apple or pineapple juice.

(Liquid Diet #4 Cont.)

> 1 cup milk
> 1 slice bread **or** 7 saltines **or** 3 graham crackers

5. 1-1/2 fruit i.e. three-quarters cup juice as in #4
   1-1/2 slices bread **or** 10 saltines **or** 4-1/2 graham crackers

6. 3/4 cup Jello
   3 saltines
   1 cup soup (diluted)

7. 1-1/2 cups soup (diluted)
   1-1/2 slices bread **or** 10 saltines **or** 7 Ritz crackers

8. 1 cup apple **or** orange juice
   1 slice bread **or** 7 saltines

9. 1 cup Metrecal
   1/2 slice toast **or** 3 graham crackers

10. 1/2 cup ice cream
    1-1/2 slices toast **or** 10 saltines

11. 1-1/2 cups 7-Up **or** Ginger Ale

NOTE: Broth or bouillon may be taken as desired.

Chapter 11 FOOT CARE

Diabetic patients have a high incidence of foot problems. This is particularly true of middle-aged and elderly persons with diabetes. This is the result of:

1. Altered resistence to infection. At times this may be associated with poorly controlled diabetes. More often it is due to a poor state of health of the skin.

2. Changes in the state of health of the skin due to:
   A. Atherosclerosis or thickening of the walls of the arteries of the lower legs and feet, resulting in poor nourishment of the skin and the tissue beneath the skin.
   B. Diabetic neuropathy or neuritis, which leads to diminished or absent pain sensation. As a result, heat, pressure sites on the toes and under surfaces of the feet, and foot ulcers are more easily overlooked. This allows for further injury of the skin, development or progression of corns and calluses or extension of existing foot ulcers.

As a result of this vulnerability of the tissues of the feet, the feet must be protected from infection and injury. This can be achieved by following these instructions in foot care.

FOOT CARE INSTRUCTIONS

1. Wash feet daily in warm water, using a mild soap. Inspect the toes and feet during gentle drying.

2. Change socks daily. Avoid garters or other constrictive bands.

3. If the skin of the feet and lower legs is dry, scaly or cracked, apply lanolin once or twice daily. If the feet tend to be moist, treat with a non-medicated talcum powder.

4. Cut the toenails straight across. If this is difficult to accomplish or if vision is poor, it is advisable to seek the services of a podiatrist.

5. Avoid sunburn.

6. Tobacco should not be used.

7. Pressure areas on toes or early degrees of ingrown toenails should be protected by pads of lamb's wool. The corner of a nail may be lifted away from the skin by continuous use of lamb's wool.

8. Many people with diabetes complain of cold feet, particularly at night. The only safe and often effective measure is to wear heavy bed socks at night.

9. Avoid the application of:
   — Medicated ointment without the advice of a physician.
   — Corn remedies.
   — Adhesive tape.
   — Heat.

10. Minor abrasions and cuts should be washed with warm water and protected by a light, dry dressing. If the injury is associated with swelling, or the cut is rather extensive, weight-bearing should be avoided. Consult with your physician or podiatrist.

11. A bruising injury of the toes or foot due to a sprain, tripping, or from a heavy object striking the toe, will cause swelling and possibly further impairment of circulation to the injured area. Therefore:
   A. Keep the foot elevated.
   B. Avoid weight-bearing.
   C. Do not use any application of either cold or heat.
   D. Consult a physician or podiatrist.

12. Always wear comfortable, roomy shoes.

13. New shoes should be broken in slowly by increasing their use by one half hour each day.

14. If there is a foot injury and weight bearing is permitted, use shoes that will not increase pressure to the injured area.

15. Athlete's foot should not be treated indiscriminately with over-the-counter medications. Consult with a physician or podiatrist about appropriate treatment measures.

SPECIAL FOOT PROBLEMS

CORNS AND CALLUSES

Calluses are areas of skin that have become thickened. Corns are hardened, localized calluses. The thickening is the result of constant rubbing by shoes against the skin of the feet. Severe degrees of corns and calluses may be due to underlying bony prominences. Pressure because of constriction or friction between adjacent toes where the skin is moist can lead to soft corns.

The treatment of corns and calluses requires regular trimming by a physician or podiatrist. If there are pressure sites, advice regarding the fitting of shoes should be requested.

If blisters or ulcers begin to develop, avoid weight-bearing and consult with your physician. At times surgery is required to correct unusual bony prominences.

Soft corns are managed by drying the web spaces between the toes and by separating the affected toes. Rubbing alcohol and non-medicated talcum powder will help to keep the skin dry. The toes can be separated by a pad of lamb's wool.

BLISTERS, INFLAMED AND SWOLLEN AREAS, ULCERS — Immediately consult a physician.

THICKENED OR DISTORTED TOENAILS — This requires the attention of a physician or podiatrist.

TO NOT APPLY HEAT LOCALLY TO A TOE OR TO THE FOOT FOR REASONS OF PAIN, INJURY OR INFECTION.

Part 4

COMPLICATIONS of DIABETES MELLITUS

Chapter 12 COMPLICATIONS OF DIABETES MELLITUS

DIABETIC KETOACIDOSIS

DEFINITION

Diabetic ketoacidosis is a complication of uncontrolled diabetes and is the result of a generalized upset in the metabolism of glucose, fats and protein in the body due to a severe reduction in insulin activity. As a result, there is a high concentration of glucose, fatty substances (fatty acids) and ketones in the blood. If untreated, characteristic signs and symptoms produced include coma.

CAUSES OF KETOACIDOSIS

Uncontrolled diabetes mellitus may result from:

1. Lack of insulin.
   A. Production low in the newly discovered diabetic.
   B. Failure to take insulin.
2. Acute stress reaction associated with:
   A. Acute infections with fever.
   B. Emotional stress.
   C. Severe pain due to injury, burn or heart attack.

Acute stress through stimulation of the nervous system causes the release of certain secretions (hormones) from the adrenal glands, as indicated on Pages 31, 101. These cause the liver to discharge sugar from the glucagon stores and to convert body protein to sugar. In addition, there is a breakdown in fat stores, freeing fatty acids. The result is a rising blood glucose and an increase in the level of fatty acids in the bloodstream. This sets the stage in the liver for ketone formation as follows:

1. The blood sugar level continues to increase, stimulating loss of body water through the kidneys as increasing amounts of sugar are discharged.

2. Fat metabolism is interrupted with accumulation of fatty acids.

3. The liver begins to form ketone substances from the fatty acids in increasing amounts, leading to the secretion of the ketones by the kidney into the urine. This is the beginning of ketoacidosis.

SYMPTOMS OF KETOACIDOSIS

As the state of ketoacidosis progresses, the early phase may reveal such symptoms as:

1. Thirst and diminishing secretion of urine.
2. Fatigue.
3. Possible loss of appetite.
4. Signs of infection of the skin, kidneys, etc.

Urine tests for glucose at this time are often 2 percent or higher and the ketone test may show small or moderate in amount of ketones present.

In the moderately advanced phase, symptoms such as:

1. Noted above.
2. More acute thirst.
3. Increased tiredness associated with weakness.
4. Nausea associated with loss of appetite.

Urine test for glucose is usually 2 percent or higher and the ketone test usually reveals a moderate or large amount of ketones present.

In the advanced phase, symptoms are:

1. As above.
2. Nausea and vomiting; abdominal pain.
3. Shortness of breath (Kussmaul respirations); sweet odor on breath.
4. Drowsiness.

The urine now reveals over 2 percent sugar and large amounts of ketones.

DIAGNOSIS OF KETOACIDOSIS

The diagnosis of ketoacidosis is made when the urine test for sugar is 2 percent or more and the ketone test of urine shows moderate or large amounts of ketones (See p. 112).

PREVENTION OF KETOACIDOSIS DURING ACUTE ILLNESS

See instructions on page 116.

DIABETIC NEURITIS

Diabetic neuritis is a disorder of nerve function. Some of the first signs are numbness and tingling in the feet or a shooting or burning pain in the lower legs. A few patients note dizziness on first rising in the morning. Impotence can also result from diabetic neuritis.

The most common form of neuritis is that involving the sensory nerves, the nerves that record sensations. This may lead to two different patterns of complaints:

1. *PAINFUL NEURITIS* — burning or stabbing pain in the lower legs and feet. This is most likely to occur at night while at rest or in bed. It is commonly accompanied by an increased sensitivity of the feet to touch or pressure. Uncontrolled diabetes frequently precedes this form of neuritis, and treatment is directed towards improved control. In older people, arteriosclerosis may lead to painful neuritis. Treatment is directed towards improving circulation and careful skin and foot care.

2. *PAINLESS NEURITIS* — is more often discovered in middle-aged persons with mild diabetes. The first symptom is usually numbness in the feet. Others discover they have lost the capacity to recognize pain — such as a woman who inched closer to the fireplace one chilly winter night. The next morning the front of her lower legs were reddened from a superficial heat burn. When painless neuritis is present it becomes mandatory that the feet be inspected every time they are washed. Under these circumstances one should not apply heat to the feet and lower legs. Careful breaking in of new shoes is a must.

3. *OTHER FORMS OF NEURITIS MAY LEAD TO:*
   A. Muscular weakness, e.g. of an eye muscle with resulting double vision; or a lower leg muscle leading to a foot drop.
   B. A marked drop in blood pressure on standing. If this occurs on rising in the morning it may cause a feeling of lightheadedness, weakness or shaking which can be confused with hypoglycemia (low blood sugar). Impotence in some males is a result of diabetic neuritis. In others it can be associated with poorly controlled diabetes. In this latter group, improved nutrition with control of diabetes can be helpful.

ATHEROSCLEROSIS

Atherosclerosis causes narrowing of arteries. It is a health problem in our western society and is seen increasingly in men after the age of 30 and women after the age of 45. The cause is unknown. However, it is recognized that persons with diabetes, high blood pressure and disorders of lipid (fat) metabolism are more prone to develop atherosclerosis. Strokes, heart attacks and poor arterial circulation in the legs are complications of atherosclerosis. Warning symptoms precede these complications. Angina, a pain in the region of the breast bone with exertion or emotional stress, should be reported. Other symptoms worth reporting to the physician are cramps in the calves of the lower legs during walking, temporary disturbances of vision or speech, dizziness, lapses of memory, and fleeting weakness or tingling in an arm or leg. The site of atherosclerosis can often be isolated by arteriography or x-rays of the arteries. When identified, these areas may be bypassed surgically. This may produce relief from the symptoms of atherosclerosis.

Young to middle aged adults with coronary arteriosclerosis and angina may be urged to lose weight if appropriate, and to follow a diet low in saturated fats and cholesterol (See p. 79).

DISORDERS OF KIDNEY FUNCTION

KIDNEY INFECTION

Some persons with diabetes are prone to have repeated infections of the kidneys. This may represent a lowered resistence to infection in the urinary tract due to the presence of too much glucose (sugar) in the urine for too long a period of time. Sugar promotes the growth of bacteria.

Repeated infections of the kidneys can cause tissue damage and interference in the function of the kidneys. Kidney infections do not always cause fever and backache. The urine must be examined for the presence of bacteria and white cells. The discovery of bacteria or white cells is an indication for a urine culture to discover the nature of the invading bacteria. In this way the appropriate use of antibiotics can be decided and the infection treated. Infections when present are best treated early. Reinfection is possible and must be watched for. Careful control of diabetes is beneficial in preventing reinfection. If reinfection is a common problem, urological examination is desirable.

DIABETIC NEPHROPATHY

It is not unusual for those who have had diabetes for many years, and who had diabetes discovered early in life, to develop persistence of albumin in the urine, puffiness of the feet, elevation in blood pressure and anemia. These findings suggest the presence of diabetic nephropathy — a condition of the kidneys due to a combination of changes. These changes are observed by microscope and consist of the presence of scar tissue resulting from kidney infections, narrowing of the small kidney arteries due to arteriosclerosis and thickening of the basement membrane. The basement membrane is a filtering membrane in the small filtering units of the kidneys called glomeruli.

As diabetic nephropathy progresses over the years it can result in uremia, or kidney failure. In recent years this condition has been treated by hemodialysis and kidney transplantation. These treatments have been used with increasing success, to correct the symptoms of chronic renal failure and hypertension. Renal transplantation was pioneered by a group at the University of Minnesota. In 1973, Dr. John Najarian of this group[1] reported that diabetics in renal failure could benefit from renal transplantation. They can develop functioning renal grafts, better control of their hypertension and greater stability of their vision. There was no difficulty regulating the blood glucose levels after transplantation even though the patients were on corticosteroids.

DIABETES AND DISORDERS OF VISION

Microangiopathy or small blood vessel disease is a complication associated with diabetes. Diabetes retinopathy is an example of microangiopathy and involves the small vessels of the inner lining or retina of the eye. Diabetic retinopathy is now the second leading cause of blindness in the United States. Before discussing diabetic retinopathy it might be well to note that there are some other less serious causes of visual disorders.

1. Blurring of vision occurs with changes in blood glucose levels. Hypoglycemia is a temporary cause of blurring of vision. Occasionally during the onset of symptomatic diabetes blurring of vision accompanies hyperglycemia or elevated blood sugar. At other times, a period of impaired vision occurs following correction of a persistently elevated blood sugar level. It is for this reason that patients are advised to wait a few weeks before having their eyes examined for glasses.

2. Cataracts which are a thickening or clouding of the lens of the eye lead to blurring of vision. There are two major forms of cataracts, both of which may be remedied by surgery. One, a metabolic cataract, develops occasionally in relation to diabetes. The other, a senile cataract which develops in elderly persons, is a much more common form.

3. Diabetic retinopathy is a degenerative condition involving the small blood vessels of the retina or inner lining of the eye. It is becoming increasingly an important cause of visual disability. About 10 percent of persons discovering the presence of diabetes after age 60 years may have retinopathy. Diabetic retinopathy is very rarely detected under the age of 20. It is diagnosed more often after age 20, and some 50 percent learning of diabetes between the ages of 30 and 60 will have retinopathy within a period of 10 years. The serious aspects of retinopathy relate to the type of retinopathy present.

    A. Background retinopathy refers to the presence of exudates or pools of serum which have leaked from the blood vessels near the retina. If this serum leaks in the region of the macula, the most sensitive seeing area of the eye, it results in impaired or even loss of vision. This is found to be a major problem in older people, and up to 40 percent with this problem can become visually handicapped.

    B. Diabetic retinopathy in younger persons is of two types generally:

        1) Non-proliferative type — indicates the presence of microaneurysms and small hemorrhages. Microaneurysms are small sac-like protrusions of the small vessel wall — when one ruptures it results in a localized spot of blood or hemorrhage beside the small blood vessel. In 3 percent of those under 30

years of age with this form of retinopathy and good vision, there may be loss of vision in five years.

2) Proliferative type of retinopathy indicates the presence of newly formed blood vessels and scar tissue. This form of retinopathy is accompanied by a) hemorrhages of blood into the vitreous or the fluid which fills the eye, b) formation of scar tissue. Complications of this process are loss of vision due to blood in the vitreous, detachment of the retina and hemorrhagic glaucoma.

Until recent years there was no way of dealing with progressive diabetic retinopathy. Then, in 1953, Dr. Jacob Poulsen[2] in Denmark reported an amazing degree of recovery from diabetic retinopathy in a young lady with diabetes whose anterior pituitary gland ceased to function. After this observation was reported, Drs. Luft and Olivecrona[3] of Sweden and others in this country, particularly Drs. Pearson and Ray,[4] began experimenting with hypophysectomy treat as a treatment of diabetic retinopathy.

Hypophysectomy, or surgical removal of the gland was found to benefit some forms of retinopathy. As an alternative to surgery, radiation of the gland has evolved as a treatment for inactivating the pituitary gland. One method of radiation developed at the Lawrence Laboratory in Berkeley, California and other laboratories employs the teletherapeutic delivery of high energy heavy ions.[5]

In recent years, hypophysectomy has been less frequently recommended because of the success often accompanying early treatment of non-proliferative retinopathy and some forms of retinopathy revealing new blood vessel formation by Argon Laser.

Argon Laser emits high energy waves that are absorbed by the hemoglobin of the red blood cells circulating in the small blood vessels. The heat developed at the areas treated cauterizes the blood vessels. Dr. Francis L'Esperance[6] of New York City and Dr. C. Zweng[7] of Palo Alto have demonstrated that the use of Argon Laser treatment can prevent many of the complications of diabetic retinopathy that lead to loss of vision. The use of Argon Laser is usually preceded by evaluation of the blood vessels by fluoresein angiography. Fluoresein is a dye, which after intravenous injection, can indicate areas of the retina requiring treatment.

Quite recently a new procedure has been introduced called vitrectomy.

This surgical procedure is being evaluated as a means for treating individuals who have suffered loss of vision due to recurrent hemorrhages into the vitreous of the eye or due to scar tissue formation in the vitreous and detachment of the retina. Vitrectomy is the surgical removal of the fluid which fills the eye. This gelatin-like material of vitreous may contain old blood and scar tissue. This diseased vitreous can now be removed by a delicate procedure involving a small rotary tube and a suction device. As the vitreous is removed it is replaced by a sterile fluid which is clear. This technique was beautifully described by Drs. W. Benson and R. Machemer of Miami, Fla. in Diabetes Forecast.* This procedure will not result in improved vision if there is disease of the optic nerve or if the retina has been severely damaged from retinopathy.

The prevention of diabetic retinopathy continues to receive much attention. In Part 1 reference was made to studies by Dr. R. Guthrie indicating the favorable influence of controlled diabetes on the appearance of basement membrane thickening in small blood vessels. Many physicians consider that control of diabetes contributes to a delay in the appearance of diabetic retinopathy.

It was also reported in Part 1 that a new hormone, somatostatin, was capable of suppressing secretion of glucagon by the alpha cells of the pancreas. This substance receives its name because it is an inhibitor of growth hormone (somatotropin) release by the pituitary gland. Removal of the pituitary gland, the source of growth hormone, sometimes has a favorable effect on the course of diabetic retinopathy. Because somatostatin inhibits release of growth hormone, it is now being investigated as a measure for the treatment of early diabetic retinopathy. Results of these studies will not be available for some time.

*Benson, W. E. and Machemer, Robt. "And the Blind Shall See." *Diabetes Forecast* May-June '75

[1] Kjellstrand, C. M., et al. (1972) Mortality and Morbidity in Diabetic Patients Accepted for Renal Transplantation. *Diabetes* 21:322.

[2] Poulsen, J. E. (1953) The Houssay Phenomenon in Man; Recovery from Retinopathy in a Case of Diabetes with Simmond's Disease. *Diabetes* 2:7.

[3] Luft, R., et al. (1955) Hypophysectomy in Man: Further Experiences in Severe Diabetes Mellitus. *British Med. Jour.* 2:752.

[4] Pearson, O. H., et al. (1964) Hypophysectomy for Treatment of Diabetic Retinopathy. *J.A.M.A.* 188:116.

[5] Lawrence, J. H., et al. (1963) Heavy particles, the Bragg Curve and Suppression of Pituitary Function in Diabetic Retinopathy. *Diabetes* 12:490.

[6] L'Esperance, F. A., Jr., (1969) The Treatment of Ophthalmic Vascular Disease by Argon Laser Photo Coagulation. *Trans. Amer. Acad. Ophthal. Otolaryngol.* 73:1077

[7] Little, H. L., et al. (1970) Argon Laser Slit-Lamp Retinal Photocoagulation. *Trans. Amer. Acad. Ophthal. Otolaryngol.* 74:85.

Part 5

OTHER ASPECTS OF LIVING WITH DIABETES MELLITUS

Chapter 13 OBESITY AND HYPERLIPIDEMIAS

OBESITY

Obesity is a source of anxiety for many people because of the associated social, health and cosmetic problems. Treatment is difficult and frequently not too successful. For this reason, many overweight people grasp at any promise of quick relief and thereby are very susceptible to fadism and quackery. The American Medical Association reports that appetite suppressants and reducing fads cost the public more than one hundred million dollars a year.

Obesity is particularly of concern for those who view it as a major health hazard. It is inappropriate, however, to view all states of obesity as health threatening. It is possible that in very early times, before the evolution of an agrarian society, the human race could not have survived without being able to put on weight. Obesity protected many races during periods of starvation. In more recent time, however, there has been increasing emphasis on the harmful effects of obesity. In 1959 the Society of Actuaries reported statistics relating overweight to a shortened life-span. According to these statistics, mortality increases considerably in relation to degree of overweight. The mortality was associated with an increased susceptibility to heart and circulatory problems, diabetes mellitus, cirrhosis of the liver and biliary tract disease. It now appears that the development of coronary artery disease in the obese is more likely in the presence of elevated blood pressure and serum cholesterol levels and a history of smoking. A continuing study sponsored by the Veterans Administration Hospital in Framingham, Mass. appears to confirm that persons with a more moderate obesity still have some risk to their health.

In an effort to separate overweight persons into groups where a change in health practices is to be encouraged, as opposed to being necessary to protect one's health, consider these factors:

1. Ideal body weight in relation to age and body size for most people is that which they had at age 18 to 20 years. Ideal body weight can be learned from Fig. 12.

2. Persons whose weight exceeds the levels considered desirable in Fig. 12 may be judged obese on inspection.

3. The degree of obesity is not particularly health threatening unless it is 20 percent over desirable weight. Thus, the desirable weight for a man over 25 years of age and 5 ft. 10 inches tall and of medium frame might be 150 pounds. Twenty percent of this weight is 30 pounds. A man weighing 180 pounds would be considered to definitely have too much weight.

DESIRABLE WEIGHTS FOR MEN
According to Height and Frame.
Ages 25 and Over.

HEIGHT (In Shoes)		Weight in Pounds (In Indoor Clothing)		
Feet	Inches	SMALL FRAME	MEDIUM FRAME	LARGE FRAME
5	2	112 - 120	118 - 129	126 - 141
5	4	118 - 126	124 - 136	132 - 148
5	6	124 - 133	130 - 143	138 - 156
5	8	132 - 141	138 - 152	147 - 166
5	10	140 - 150	146 - 160	155 - 174
6	0	148 - 158	154 - 170	164 - 184
6	2	156 - 167	162 - 180	173 - 194
6	4	164 - 175	172 - 190	182 - 204

DESIRABLE WEIGHTS FOR WOMEN
According to Height and Frame.
Ages 25 and Over

HEIGHT (In Shoes)		Weight in Pounds (In Indoor Clothing)		
Feet	Inches	SMALL FRAME	MEDIUM FRAME	LARGE FRAME
4	10	92 - 98	96 - 107	104 - 119
5	0	96 - 104	101 - 113	109 - 125
5	2	102 - 110	107 - 119	115 - 131
5	4	108 - 116	113 - 126	121 - 138
5	6	114 - 123	120 - 135	129 - 146
5	8	122 - 131	128 - 143	137 - 154
5	10	130 - 140	136 - 151	145 - 163
6	0	138 - 148	144 - 159	153 - 173

Note: Prepared by the Metropolitan Life Insurance Co.

FIG. 12

Much more needs to be known about the causes of obesity before specific recommendations can be developed for its treatment. For now it may be helpful to note the following:

1. Obesity occurs when the intake of calories (food) continues to exceed the expenditure of or burning up of calories by various body activities.

2. One form of obesity begins in childhood. When it is first evident during infancy, it may be the result of overfeeding and the development of many more fat cells than would normally form in conjunction with an average food intake. Though this may not be a particularly harmful form of obesity, obesity appearing during childhood or adolescence may lead to health problems. It is often a reflection of environmental influences which should be discouraged. These influences may be too much eating of high caloric food, too much snacking, large meals and little physical activity. Eating patterns established in these early years become habits and habits are hard to change. Emotional stresses may magnify the problem. Persons with obesity present since childhood need to recognize that they must turn from the old way and develop a new way of eating. This may be aided by such supportive dietary services as TOPS or Weight Watchers, which recognize the value of group participation in dietary programs for weight reduction.

3. Obesity developing after the age of 20 or 25 years may not be due to any real increase in caloric intake. It may instead be the result of adopting a more sedentary manner of living. This has been precipitated for many by urban living and the availability of the automobile. Some scientists report that aging is accompanied by a decrease in caloric requirements — and that obesity can develop even when food intake remains constant.

4. The treatment of obesity is **successful when:**
   A. The daily caloric intake is reduced. These calories may be supplied by the use of three, four or five scheduled feedings per day. High caloric foods and unplanned snacking between meals must be omitted.
   B. Sedentary habits give way to a regular program or adequate physical activity.
   C. Emotional strain is reduced. Emotional stresses lead to over-eating and obesity aggravates one's emotional state.

5. Appetite suppressant pills have not helped in the control of excessive appetite and some have been found to be toxic, eg. rainbow pills being toxic to the heart and causing low levels of serum potassium.

The methods recommended for the treatment of moderate obesity are:

1. Reduction in caloric intake. The number of calories will vary according to the degree of weight loss desirable, activity, age and sex.

2. Adoption of a new eating pattern that can be regularly followed, avoiding faddist diets.

3. A regular program of increased physical activity.

4. A medical examination to exclude some of the infrequent medical causes of excessive weight.

5. Measures to deal with the emotional factors which contribute to or are a consequence of obesity.

In cases of extreme obesity, severe therapeutic measures may be necessary. Examples of such measures are fasting, and a surgical procedure short-circuiting ingested food, from where it arrives in the upper small bowel into the lower end of the small bowel, i.e. a by-pass of the ileum.

Fasting leads to dehydration, a decrease in body content of certain salts, a rise in blood uric acid, a drop in blood pressure and some depletion of body protein. For these reasons, fasting should not be prolonged, and should be done under continuous medical supervision. The fast should be modified by the free intake of fluids, the intake of a small amount of protein foods, and supplementary vitamins and salts, including potassium. Fasting is not recommended for patients with gout, liver disease, or cardio-vascular disorders. Fasting produces loss of appetite and excessive ketones in the body.

Surgical by-pass of the small bowel has the attraction of permitting the intake of food, even the large amounts to which many have become accustomed. However, the procedure often has an undesirable effect, chronic diarrhea, and may be harmful to the liver.

The above procedures are described but not necessarily recommended. The material is presented to be informative. Before considering either procedure there should be a full exploration of the merits and the possible adverse side effects with experienced physicians.

HYPERLIPIDEMIAS AND HYPERLIPOPROTEINEMIAS

In recent years a group of metabolic disorders, known as hyperlipoproteinemias, have been identified that are associated with higher than normal levels of blood fats (lipids). Increased levels of cholesterol and triglycerides in the blood plasma are referred to as hyperlipidemias. Many persons with diabetes have elevated plasma levels of cholesterol and triglycerides.

Blood lipids, because they are insoluble in such watery solutions as blood plasma, must be transported in a special way. This is accomplished through the lipids being linked with certain proteins in the liver to form complex substances referred to as lipoproteins. Different forms of lipoproteins exist. One helps carry fats absorbed from the intestinal tract to body tissues. Another important one is formed in the liver by the combination of ingested carbohydrate with fatty acids and proteins. The lipoproteins carry cholesterol and triglycerides through the blood to muscle and adipose tissue. The triglycerides are stored as body fat so that they can later be available as an energy source.

Elevated blood plasma levels of lipoproteins are referred to as **hyperlipoproteinemias**. Hyperlipoproteinemias may occur as a primary disorder, because of the inheritance of certain genetic factors, or they may be a complication of alcoholism, uncontrolled diabetes, hypothyroidism, or diseases of the liver, kidneys or pancreas.

Two of the inherited forms of hyperlipoproteinemia are quite rare. One of these is called Type I and is due to a lack of a blood fat clearing factor. It is treated by restricting the dietary intake of fat. The other, Type II, is accompanied by a very high plasma cholesterol. Treatment requires the elimination of foods from the diet that contain cholesterol and the use of certain medications.

The more common lipoproteinemias, Types III, IV and V have high plasma triglyceride levels due to a genetic disorder resulting in elevated plasma triglyceride levels in combination with varying levels of plasma cholesterol. Many persons first learn of these problems after visiting a dermatologist for the investigation of small, discreet, elevated, pale-colored swellings of the skin. Others are found to have an elevated plasma triglyceride level when studied for diabetes, obesity or heart disease. When the familial forms of hyperlipoproteinemia are discovered, other family members should be periodically tested. This permits early discovery and treatment and protection from arteriosclerosis.

The majority of persons with Type IV hyperlipoproteinemia (the most common form) are overweight. With the restriction of caloric intake and weight loss, the problem can often be controlled. Such a diet will reflect less carbohydrate intake, which decreases the amount of lipoprotein formed. On occasions the physician may wish to add such medications as clofibrate (Atromid-S) and nicotinic acid, which help to decrease the production of and to clear triglyceride from the serum.

Diets low in cholesterol, low in animal fats (saturated fats) and high in polyunsaturated fats are recommended for those with abnormal elevations of plasma cholesterol. Lists of such foods can be obtained from one's physician.

Chapter 14 MENSTRUATION CONTRACEPTION — PREGNANCY

Diabetes in women most often is discovered after age 40. Therefore this discussion will be of interest to only a relatively small number of diabetic women. The subjects to be reviewed will have particular interest according to the age of the reader. Some with the onset of diabetes before the menarche* will find the onset of menstruation delayed, even beyond fifteen years of age. Later with approaching maturity, interest may turn to the influences of diabetes on pregnancy. It is appropriate to be knowledgeable about the following questions: is pregnancy possible and how does it affect diabetes; how does the diabetes influence the course of pregnancy; is the health of the baby affected in any way; and what are the baby's chances of developing diabetes?

With maturity, contraception and family planning are of more immediate concern. Counseling is encouraged in these subjects. In this way not only will decisions be made concerning the advisability and desirability of pregnancy, but diabetes management programs will be discussed, as well as the advantages of the contributions of the obstetricians and pediatricians who are members of the diabetic pregnancy management team.

*Menarche — the onset of menstruation.

The delay in the beginning of menstruation which occurs in some with juvenile onset diabetes, nearly always is followed by the appearance of menstruation. Initially the menses may occur irregularly every two or three months. Regularity is established eventually in most women. Until the latter happens, there will be some thoughts about the possibility of infertility. Infertility among well nourished and otherwise healthy young women is of about the same incidence as it is among non-diabetic women. Infertility during periods of poorly controlled diabetes affords such persons an opportunity to re-establish controlled diabetes before considering pregnancy.

Contraception is achieved with varying degrees of success relative to the measures used:

1. Abstinence from intercourse during the ovulatory period is referred to as the rhythm method. Ovulation occurs any time from 12 to 16 days before the next menses of a 28 day cycle. The rhythm method requires abstinence for seven days prior to and seven days after the 4-day ovulatory period, or a total of 18 days. If this is not acceptable, then it can be used in conjunction with such prophylactic measures as condoms, diaphragms and vaginal creams or vaginal foams. These measures are the least dependable.

2. Oral contraceptives.
Oral contraceptive pills consist of certain quantities of female hormones. These are two forms of pills — combined and sequential. The combined pills are the most effective in preventing pregnancy. These hormones initiate certain responses in relation to insulin secretion and action in the body comparable to those occurring during pregnancy. In either case there can be aggravation of early or undetected diabetes. Therefore, caution is suggested concerning their use in one with a strong family history of diabetes or who showed mild diabetes during a previous pregnancy. There is no reason, however, for those with insulin-dependent diabetes not to use them, although an adjustment in insulin dosage may be required.

Oral contraceptives are convenient and effective. They should be taken under medical supervision and in conjunction with periodic breast and pelvic examinations. Women with a history of disorders of blood coagulation or vein problems may find another mode of contraception preferable. Oral contraceptives may aggravate migraine headaches, occasionally cause stomach distress or be followed by a period of amenorrhea, or absence of menstruation, when their use is discontinued.

3. Intrauterine devices.

These mechanical devices are widely and effectively used by women throughout the world. They may, on occasion, cause or be associated with an inflammatory reaction. Pelvic infections are a potential danger in young persons using I.U.D.'s in association with poorly controlled diabetes.

4. Surgical measures. Surgical measures such as tubal ligation or vasectomy are requested by and performed for those who for medical or other reasons have a need or desire to prevent future pregnancies.

Contraception has not only made effective family planning a fact, but it has permitted some to approach marriage and reproduction with a different set of values and attitudes. Many women in their child-bearing years are conscious of a need for population control. Others feel it may be a greater contribution to adopt a child than to bear children. Some with diabetes have concluded it might be better not to chance having offspring who might develop diabetes. Dr. Priscilla White has found from her studies that diabetes is more common in the children of diabetic mothers than in the children of non-diabetic mothers. This is not so for the children of diabetic fathers.

When pregnancy does happen, the early stages of fetal development may be affected adversely by poorly controlled diabetes. Therefore, a planned pregnancy should be preceded by an adequate degree of controlled diabetes. While pregnant it is important to have regular examinations by both the physician managing the diabetes and the obstetrician. The eventual outcome is dependent on maintaining controlled diabetes, prevention of excessive accumulations of fluid, control of blood pressure. The patient must 1) adhere to a measured diet; 2) make regular tests of the urine for glucose and ketones; 3) keep a record of the test results and hypoglycemic reactions; and 4) report unusual stresses or loss of control of diabetes. In this way it is possible to keep abreast of changing insulin requirements which often characterize diabetes during pregnancy. Other complications such as frequent or severe headaches, bleeding, swelling of the feet and ankles, or sudden weight gain should also be reported. During the course of pregnancy it may be necessary to reduce the intake of table salt and take diuretics (medicine to increase the output of urine) to control the retention of excessive amounts of body fluids. The incidence of miscarriage is increased with pregnancy complicated by the presence of diabetes. Cigarette smoking may also have an adverse effect. Chronic use of alcohol and drug abuse have been proven to adversely affect the health and development of the baby.

The last weeks of pregnancy require more frequent medical examinations to assess the state of diabetic control, blood pressure levels, kidney function, and weight control. In some parts of Europe it is common to hospitalize those with diabetes who are about seven months pregnant. In either case, the stability of the pregnancy is assessed by the measurement of estriol in 24-hour urine collections. As long as these levels are adequate, the pregnancy is continued towards the anticipated delivery date. Some physicians, particularly when their cases are under constant supervision in the hospital, continue to full term and a pelvic delivery. Many other physicians plan delivery by the 37th week of pregnancy, by inducing labor or cesarean section. The delivery date is selected by studying samples of amniotic fluid drawn from the uterus. The fluid is analyzed to assess whether the fetus is mature enough to maintain adequate respiratory function following delivery. It is recommended that the infant be immediately cared for by a pediatrician following delivery. The infant requires careful study and management the first few days until its respiratory function is established and its nutritional requirements are being met. It is usual to achieve the latter by bottle feedings.

Pregnancy is rarely followed by any evidence of aggravation of juvenile diabetes. However, adults with mild diabetes may find that pregnancy is followed by a degree of diabetes that requires more attention to treatment measures. At times there is aggravation of diabetic retinopathy during pregnancy, followed by some degree of improvement after delivery. Pregnancy has been successfully completed in many women demonstrating signs of impaired kidney function.

Where a team of physicians (internist, obstetrician and pediatrician) interested in diabetes work in conjunction with experienced nursing personnel, fetal survival may reach 90 percent. Ten percent or more of pregnancies are not successfully terminated due to miscarriage, death of the infant in utero, or death following delivery. In the latter instance the causes may be due to prematurity, respiratory distress syndrome, congenital abnormalities or other rare conditions. A few years ago it was common for many hospitals to report no more than a 50 to 75 percent survival of infants from diabetic pregnancies. The survival figures have improved for many reasons, among them, management by a team of physicians, better management of diabetes during pregnancy, improved diuretics, better methods for planning the time of delivery, antibiotics, determination of salt and water needs, exchange transfusions and the use of incubators.

Chapter 15   EMPLOYABILITY
INSURANCE – LONGEVITY

EMPLOYMENT AND EMPLOYABILITY

Employability may be of great concern to one with a chronic health problem. Will a prospective employer be sympathetic towards the job applicant with diabetes? Is a particular industry suitable for a diabetic worker? Which professions are open to diabetic persons? Can diabetes jeopardize opportunities for promotion or for inclusion in health insurance programs?

A 1957 survey of the American Diabetes Association (ADA) reported nearly thirty percent of small and large companies were reluctant to employ diabetic people. Such policies, when rigidly adhered to, are inappropriate and the authors agree with the 1965 World Health Organization statement that, "The restrictions are purely negative and are based on prejudice or ill-informed opinion about the effect of diabetes on a person's working ability or capacity." WHO reports further, "This is bound up with the mistake of failing to distinguish between mild cases and cases under appropriate medical control on the one hand, and uncooperative, uncontrolled cases on the other." Further, the mild or well-controlled diabetic worker may even be more dependable because of his more regular living pattern, regular health check-ups and the desire to remain at the job. He is a good employment risk. On the other hand, the Committee on Employment of the ADA recommends that poorly controlled or uncooperative diabetic persons should be refused employment. The young diabetic anticipating employment should seek the counseling and guidance of well-informed persons before entering into job training or continuing his professional education.

Many professions are open to the diabetic, particularly in education, in the ministry, and in nursing and other health careers. He may experience difficulty entering medicine, but less difficulty going into dentistry and law. The young diabetic will probably not be able to enter the armed service academies. Many diabetic athletes continued their careers — notably, Bill Talbert and Hal Richardson in tennis, Cooley O'Brien in football, Ron Santo in baseball, and Bobby Clark in hockey, with stardom achieved in each instance. Business, horticulture and many government positions are among other attractive possibilities.

Some individuals developing diabetes during the course of their employment may lose their jobs. Others, when it becomes necessary to use insulin for the treatment of their diabetes, must be prepared to accept a shift to a less sensitive position. It is not a good health practice to substitute anti-diabetic oral tablets for insulin for too long, merely to continue one's job, if this results in poorly controlled diabetes. Those who are subject to the more severe symptoms of hypoglycemia should not work at unsafe heights, work around moving machinery, or continue in positions where they may jeopardize others. Diabetics using insulin cannot fly aircraft, operate locomotives or drive buses. They should probably not go to sea. There must be some acceptance of these limitations and, of course, a responsibility for the welfare of others. The individual's performance may affect the future employment of other diabetics. It may be best to seek other employment if the job is conducive to irregular hours, unusual variations in physical activity and undependable eating hours. Less than ten percent of the known diabetics in the United States are disabled or unemployed. Nearly forty percent are actively employed. The remainder are housewives or retired.

INSURANCE FOR DIABETICS

Insurance programs are generally difficult to develop for diabetics. Many, through their employment or the Veterans Administration, have been able to qualify for group hospital and indemnity insurance programs, and in some states Blue Cross will issue insurance coverage to an individual with diabetes. In other parts of the country there may be a waiting period of up to 12 months. Most individually issued programs have a rider on the policy for diabetes and related problems, which excludes these conditions. Life insurance is obtainable from some companies, frequently only by payment of a higher premium.

Group health insurance now is available through the Diabetes Group Insurance Trust. For the Trust to operate in all states, membership in the American Diabetes Association is required. Enrollment dates for this program are available from the American Diabetes Association, 1 West 48th Street, New York, N.Y., 10020. (Telephone 212-541-4310.) It is understood that once a policy is issued, it cannot be cancelled by the insuring company, nor may the rates be increased.

Since early 1974 individual life insurance at standard rates, without medical examination, has been available to diabetics between the ages of 15 and 65 years, who are members of the American Diabetes Association. Two plans are offered to members through Counselor Service of Philadelphia, Pa. One plan is paid-up insurance at age 65, while the other is a twenty payment life plan. Both plans are available in amounts from $5,000 to $25,000, depending upon the age of the applicant. To qualify, the applicant must have developed diabetes since 1958, be under medical control with periodic examinations by a physician, be free of symptoms of cardiovascular or kidney disease, and be a member of the ADA or of an affiliate, chapter, branch or unit.

LONGEVITY AND DIABETES

There are more early deaths in the diabetic population than in the non-diabetic population. This can, in part, be attributed to a higher incidence of high blood pressure, coronary artery disease and kidney disease. Age of onset and duration of diabetes as well as prolonged periods of uncontrolled diabetes have a significant influence. It is of interest to review the experience of the Joslin Clinic, Boston, from 1897 to 1957 in relation to a study on "Duration of Life Subsequent to the Onset of Diabetes among 18,055 Deceased Diabetics". Before the introduction of insulin, those with onset of diabetes at age 10 could expect to live up to 3 years, at age 30 up to 5 years, and at age 50 up to 8 years. After the introduction of insulin the life expectancy for those with onset before age 30 was doubled.

During the 1940's, with the introduction of antibiotics, the duration of life for those with onset of diabetes before age 20 again increased significantly. As a result of improved anesthesia, surgical techniques and many other advances in medicine, through the 1960's life expectancy for white male diabetics was greater than 62 years; for white females it was more than 66 years. That one with D.M. can live far beyond these averages was demonstrated by the noted British physician, diabetic specialist and researcher, Dr. Robert Daniel Lawrence. Shortly after his discharge from the army following World War I and while in his late 20's, he was discovered to have diabetes. This was two years before the discovery of insulin by Drs. Fredrich Banting and Charles Best in Toronto, Canada. Dr. Lawrence managed to get by until insulin became available, and thereafter was able to live a most productive and satisfying life. Most of these years were used in research, practicing medicine and contributing to the welfare of diabetic people. He was a co-founder of the British Diabetes Association. He died in 1969 at the age of 76 years.

Chapter 16   TRAVEL SUGGESTIONS

Persons with insulin-dependent diabetes must plan ahead before going on vacations, short trips, or special outings. A change in routine can alter diabetes control. It is possible to anticipate which changes in routine will have an effect on diabetes. Certain aspects of the daily diabetic program can be adjusted to accommodate these changes, such as diet, insulin dose and activities. In addition, one must prepare for emergencies by having an additional supply of needles, syringes, materials for the prevention and treatment of hypoglycemia, and extra food. Special precautions may be required for the care of insulin.

It is always important for the diabetic to wear an identification tag or bracelet showing name, address, and medical problem along with any other significant information. This is even more important when traveling. This will assist in the handling of the diabetic who cannot communicate well, to insure early and appropriate medical care. A notation on the tag may indicate "refer to wallet card" for more complete instructions.

While traveling, have extra supplies close at hand. Luggage can go astray. Insulin and other supplies should be kept in a suitcase or other bag which you keep with you at all times, so that it is always readily available when needed. Insulin is quite stable at room temperature. As extreme temperatures are damaging, these effects should be avoided by using an insulated container.

EXTRA SUPPLIES SHOULD INCLUDE:
1. Insulin
2. Needles and syringes (disposable are usually satisfactory)
3. Urine test materials
4. Instant glucose, sugar cubes, glucagon
5. Food
   Graham crackers, saltines
   Cheese
   Certain dehydrated foods
   Fresh fruit
   Sandwiches
   Fruit juices

ADDITIONAL ITEMS FOR HIKING

Candy bars
Dehydrated foods, fruits, vegetables, soups
Beef Jerky
Granola (See p. 169), cocoa mix (See p. 153)

DIET ADJUSTMENTS WHEN TRAVELING

Experienced dieters should be able to estimate amounts and kinds of foods for most meals.

INSULIN-DEPENDENT DIABETICS

1. Inactivity imposed by air or car travel. Introduce one of the following:
   a. Decrease carbohydrate intake 10 to 15 percent at meals.
   b. Omit an afternoon or evening snack.
   c. Arrange exercise periods mid-morning or mid-afternoon.
   d. If persistent glucosuria results, then an adjustment of the insulin dose may be necessary.
2. Excess physical activity
   a. Use extra feedings while hiking, even as often as every three hours on backpacking trips.
   b. Decrease a.m. insulin dose if so advised after counseling with one's physician.
   c. Sip fruit juice or carbonated sweet drinks during periods of unusual physical activity.

DIABETICS MANAGED BY DIET OR DIET AND AN ORAL DIABETIC TABLET:

It is unusual for those with this milder form of diabetes to lose control of their diabetes as a result of periods of inactivity or because of eating meals away from home. When away on a trip or eating with friends in their home or in restaurants, it is well to continue diet estimation. There may be occasions when this is impractical. If so, do not be frustrated or upset by the experience. It is best that people participate in daily living experiences and enjoy their involvements. Occasional dietary indiscretions do not cause uncontrolled diabetes.

TIME ZONE CHANGES

Air travel allows for quick passage from one time zone to another. Insulin-dependent diabetics are required to make adjustments in time of insulin injection and hours of eating as they accommodate to a new time schedule. This is not too difficult when traveling into an adjacent time zone. If the time spread is three or more hours, more specific planning is required. To assist in this planning the following suggestions are offered:

1. If there is a total time change of 2 to 3 hours on the day of travel, adhere to the usual daily schedule, i.e. lunch four hours after breakfast and dinner five hours after lunch. (Do not follow meal hours of new time zone.) The following day begin breakfast one hour earlier if going west, one hour later if going east, then your usual breakfast hour, in the new time zone. Again, space the meals as indicated above.
The next day follow the routine meal hours in accordance with the time zone.

2. If there is a total time change of 4 to 6 hours, begin two hours earlier if going west or two hours later if going east the day after arrival. Again, space the meals by the usual interval. The following day can be started one hour off your usual meal hours existing in the new time zone.

3. Persons using 20 units or less insulin may find it convenient to have a light meal at the dinner hour of the time zone when traveling east, followed by a substantial bed-time snack, i.e. two snacks rather than a later meal. A snack should be eaten if there is going to be a delay in receiving the next meal.

FEDERAL AVIATION ADMINISTRATION SPECIFICATIONS FOR INITIAL EVALUATION ABNORMAL CARBOHYDRATE METABOLISM

It is of primary importance that a good baseline be established for airmen seeking medical certification when there is an indication of disturbance of carbohydrate metabolism. When prior clinical information exists (hospital records, laboratory reports, out-patient resumes, etc.) this should be submitted. When the prior information submitted includes data required below, the tests need not be updated if no more than 90 days old at the time of examination. Actual electro-cardiographic tracings should be forwarded with the evaluation report.

1. General medical history, complaints.

2. Family and personal history relative to diabetes.

3. Height and weight with explanation of any recent changes in weight.

4. Ophthalmoscopic examination.

5. Vibration sense of the extremities.

6. Cardiovascular examination:
   A. History specific for cardiovascular disease.
   B. Blood pressure (brachial arteries; sitting)
   C. Circulatory efficiency in extremities.
   D. Standard 12-lead resting electrocardiogram.
   E. Double Master's exercise electrocardiogram (unless medically contraindicated; protocol attached).
   F. Blood lipid determination (total cholesterol and triglycerides).

7. Report of chest x-ray.

8. Urinalysis for specific gravity, albumin, sugar and acetone.

9. Statement concerning present need for insulin or other hypoglycemic medication for maintenance of control. If medication has previously been required for control of carbohydrate metabolism, specify types and date that latest medication was discontinued.*

10. Blood glucose determination.
    A. If a prior "diagnostic" glucose tolerance test (GTT) has been made, the results should be submitted along with current fasting and 2-hour postprandial blood sugar test results (with urine sugar and acetone findings).
    B. If no prior GTT diagnostic for diabetes, a current GTT should be submitted (3-hour acceptable, 5-hour preferred).

In all blood sugar testing the following information should be furnished in addition to the numerical measurement:

1. Applicant preparation and test load (see below — GTT).

2. Nature of sample (plasma or whole blood).

3. Test method with notation as to the laboratory's "normal" value and whether correction factors have already been incorporated to make readings equivalent to whole venous blood.

Blood sugar tests should be specific (true blood glucose), such as the Somogyi-Nelson or Autoanalyzer. The Folin-Wu is non-specific. Values obtained from capillary blood (as by finger prick) can be converted roughly to "true" glucose values (whole venous blood) by subtracting 30 mg. per 100 ml. Autoanalyzer results are usually plasma glucose levels, which generally are 25 mg. per 100 ml. higher than whole venous blood.

*IMPORTANT NOTE: Certification will be considered *only* if adequate control can be accomplished and maintained without use of hypoglycemic drugs. If use of medication has only recently been discontinued, control is to be demonstrated by fasting and 2-hour postprandial blood sugar tests taken at 30-day intervals during a 90-day period. Prior studies may be acceptable. Urine sugars a.c. and h.s. are helpful.

A postprandial blood sample should be drawn 2 hours following ingestion of 100 grams of carbohydrate (loading dose). This may be accomplished by a solution containing 100 grams of glucose, by one of the commercial preparations containing an equivalent load, or where intolerance or nausea is anticipated, by a meal such as the following:

Banana, 8 ozs. cereal, 2 slices white bread with butter
8 ozs. milk and 4 ozs. orange juice

A glucose tolerance test conducted for FAA medical certification purposes will follow these guidelines:

1. For 3 days before examination, the applicant will have eaten a full diet containing 250-300 grams of carbohydrates daily. Physical activity should not be curtailed during this period.

2. Birth control pills, thiazide diuretics, steroids and other drugs which may alter carbohydrate metabolism (including large doses of aspirin or nicotinic acid) should be avoided.

3. Applicant fasts after midnight preceding the day of the test (8-16 hrs.)

4. Fasting blood and urine specimens are obtained (preferably in the A.M.)

5. A loading dose of no more than 100 grams of glucose is ingested (water load should not be excessive).

6. Blood and urine glucose are determined at 30 minutes, one hour, two hours and three hours after ingestion of the loading dose. (4 and 5-hour samples are helpful but not required).

Part 6

RECIPES FOR THE DIABETIC

Recipes for the diabetic

APPETIZERS and BEVERAGES

CHEESE-OLIVE PUFFS

1/4 lb. sharp cheddar, swiss or Roquefort cheese, grated 112 grams
1/2 stick soft butter . . . . 56 grams
1/2 cup sifted flour . . . . 56 grams
1/4 tsp. salt . . . . free
1/2 tsp. paprika . . . . free

Blend cheese and butter and add rest of ingredients. Wrap 1 tsp. of it around olive. Chill.
Can be made two days ahead and left in refrigerator.
Bake at 400° for 12 to 15 minutes when ready to serve.

Divide total CPF by number of puff balls to get CPF per puff ball.

Total recipe = C-44; P-32; F-84

WATER CHESTNUTS ROLLED IN BACON

1/2 water chestnut . . . . 3 grams
1/3 strip bacon . . . . 3 grams

Halve each chestnut and roll in 1/3 strip of bacon and stick together with toothpick. Refrigerate. Broil for 3 minutes when ready to serve.

Total recipe = C-1; P-1; F-1

Exchange: 1 snack is free.
3 snacks = 1 fat

MILK SHAKE VARIATIONS

BASE:
1/2 cup ice milk .... 120 grams
1/2 cup skim milk .... 120 grams

VARIATIONS: .... These may be added
1 tsp. cocoa   without changing the
OR Nutmeg, few grains   value of the recipe.
OR Vanilla (1/8 tsp)

Total recipe = C-19; P-7; F-3
Exchange: 1 recipe = 1 milk (2%) + 1/2 fruit
1/2 recipe = 1 fruit + 1/2 meat

ADDITIONAL VARIATIONS

Add Banana, 1/2 small .... Total recipe = C-30; P-7; F-3
Exchange: 1 recipe = 1 fruit + 1-1/2 milk (2%)
1/2 recipe = 1 fruit + 1/2 milk
Add Strawberries 1/2 cup .... Total recipe = C-22; P-7; F-3
Exchange: 1 recipe = 1 fruit + 1 milk
Add fruit flavored frozen concentrate (diluted) 1/2 cup   120 grams
Total recipe = C-33; P-7; F-3
Exchange: 1 recipe = 2 fruit + 1 milk
1/2 recipe = 1 fruit + 1/2 milk

MINDERHOUT'S COCOA PACKETS

6 tbsp. powdered skim milk
1 tbsp. cocoa
2 saccharin tablets (or powdered sweetener to taste)

Add this mixture to 1 cup hot water for cocoa. 184 calories. This can be mixed up in individual packets and carried for backpacking, skiing or anytime a hot drink would come in handy!

1 cup = C-16; P-10; F-10

Exchange: 1 cup = 1 fruit, 1/2 meat, 1 fat & 1/2 milk

LIZ' "ORANGE JULIUS"

1 egg	50 grams
1/2 cup orange juice (fresh or frozen)	100 grams
Scant 1/2 cup vanilla ice cream	75 grams

Blend egg in blender until thick and frothy. Add orange juice and blend well. Add ice cream and blend again. Makes one large serving — for special occasions. Can pour over ice if desired.

Total recipe = C-28; P-9; F-15

Exchange: One serving equals — 1 fruit, 1½ whole milk, 1 meat.

ORANGE COOLER*

1 (12 oz.) can Diet Shasta Creme Soda	
1 cup unsweetened orange juice	
1 tbsp. lemon juice	free
Sugar substitute to taste	free

Combine all ingredients and pour over ice in tall glasses. Makes 2 servings.

Total recipe = C-28; P-0; F-0
1/2 recipe = C-14; P-0; F-0
1/3 recipe = C-9; P-0; F-0

Exchange: 1/2 recipe = 1½ fruit
1/3 recipe = 1 fruit

2 FRUIT — LIME COOLER*

1 (12 oz.) can Diet Shasta Lemon-Lime	free
1/2 cup chopped fresh pineapple	66 grams
1 cup chopped cantaloupe	240 grams
2 tbsp. lemon juice	free
Dash salt	free

Whirl all ingredients together in blender until smooth. Makes 2½ cups.

Total recipe = C-27; P-0; F-0
1/2 recipe = C-14; P-0; F-0
1/5 recipe = C-5; P-0; F-0
(1/2 cup)

Exchange: 1/2 recipe = 1½ fruit
1/5 recipe (1/2 cup) = 1/2 fruit

*Used by permission of
Shasta Beverage Company

```
──────────── GINGER PEACH DREAM* ────────────
```

1 (12 oz.) can Diet Shasta Ginger Ale . . . . free
1½ cups chopped fresh peaches
1/4 tsp. powdered ginger . . . . free
2 tbsp. lemon juice . . . . free
1/2 tsp. artificial liquid sweetener . . . . free
dash salt . . . . free

Whirl all ingredients together in blender until partially smooth. Serve well chilled or over ice. Makes 4 cups.

Total recipe = C-24; P-0; F-0
1/2 recipe = C-12; P-0; F-0
1/4 recipe = C-6; P-0; F-0

Exchange: 1/2 recipe = 1 fruit
1/4 recipe = 1/2 fruit

*Used by permission of Shasta Beverage Company

SALADS and DRESSING

```
──────────── COTTAGE CHEESE SALAD ────────────
```

1/4 tsp. cinnamon . . . . free
1 cup prepared whipped topping
1 pkg. orange diet gelatin . . . . free
1/2 pint cottage cheese
1 can (10½ oz.) w.p. Mandarin oranges (drained)

Combine, refrigerate until thickened, and serve.
Variation: use lime diet gelatin and w.p. pineapple (8½ oz. can, drained). (use the same values)

Total recipe = C-24; P-34; F-16
1/6 recipe = C-4; P-6; F-3

Exchange: 1/6 recipe = 1/2 fruit
and 1/2 meat

COLE SLAW AND DRESSING

2 tbsp. mayonnaise . . . . 30 grams
1/2 tbsp. vinegar (or to taste) . . . . free
Salt & pepper to taste . . . . free
Sugar substitute to taste . . . . free
3 cups shredded cabbage . . . . 300 grams

Yields 6 (1/2 cup) servings.   Total recipe = C-15; P-0; F-26
Mix first 4 ingredients to taste.   Each serving = C-2; P-0; F-4
Pour over cabbage, stir and serve.

Exchange: Each 1/2 cup serving = 1 Veg. and 1 fat.

PIQUANT DRESSING*

1½ cups tomato juice
1½ cups water
3/4 cup liquid pectin   Boil tomato juice and water. Add
1/2 cup red wine vinegar   liquid pectin. Cool. Add the rest
1/4 cup tarragon vinegar   of the ingredients. Shake before
3/4 tsp. salt   using.
1/2 tsp. dry mustard
1/2 tsp. onion juice
1½ tsp. liquid artificial sweetener

VINAIGRETTE DRESSING*

2½ cups water
1 cup liquid pectin
6 tbsp. red wine vinegar
6 tbsp. tarragon vinegar   Boil water. Add liquid pectin.
1/2 tsp. dry mustard   Cool. Add the rest of the ingredi-
1/4 tsp. pepper   ents. Shake before using.
few grains of thyme
1½ tsp. liquid sucaryl
3/4 tsp. onion juice

ZERO DRESSING*

3½ cups tomato juice
1/4 tsp. salt
1/4 tsp. pepper   Mix ingredients
1/2 tsp. onion juice
2 tbsp. lemon juice

*The value of these dressings is: C-0; P-0; F-0

These dressings are used by permission of the Dietary Department, Good Samaritan Hospital & Medical Center.

ENTREES

CORNED BEEF HASH*

1 slice (4"x3"x1/2") cooked corned beef . . . . 75 grams
1 small potato, boiled . . . . 75 grams
1 tsp. onion, minced . . . . free
1 egg, poached
1 tbsp. chili sauce . . . . free
salt & pepper to taste . . . . free

Chop beef and potato and onion together to desired consistency. Add salt and pepper. Brown in hot skillet. Serve with egg and chili sauce.

Total recipe = C-14; P-29; F-14

Exchange: Total recipe = 1 bread, 3 meat, 1 fat
1/2 recipe = 1/2 bread, 1½ meat, 1/2 fat

*Used by permission of Doubleday & Co., *Diabetic Menus, Meals and Recipes*, by Betty M. West.

CREAMED CHIPPED BEEF ON TOAST

2 tbsp. butter . . . . 30 grams
2 or 3 slices mushrooms . . . . free
4 oz. chipped beef, torn in pieces . . . . 120 grams
4 tsp. flour . . . . 12 grams
Dash onion powder . . . . free
1 cup skim milk . . . . 240 grams
2 slices bread . . . . 60 grams

In medium saucepan, saute mushrooms in butter until tender. Stir in flour and onion powder until smooth. Add milk and cook, stirring constantly until sauce is thick.

Add beef — cook until warmed. Toast bread, pour above mixture over toast; top with parsley sprig if desired.

Total recipe = C-52; P-50; F-33
Each serving = C-26; P-25; F-17

Exchange: Total recipe = 2½ bread, 3½ meat, 1 milk and 1/2 fat
1/2 recipe = 1 bread, 1 milk, 1½ meat and 1 fat.

JON MACETTI (meat and noodle dish)

1 lb. ground beef
1/2 lb. ground pork
3 medium onions
1 small green pepper, chopped
1/2 lb. noodles, cooked
2 cans tomato soup
1 small package Velveeta type cheese, grated
2 tsp. salt

Brown meat, onions, and green pepper in fat until brown. Add salt. Cook noodles in boiling salted water about 20 minutes. Drain, add to meat mixture with grated cheese and mix all together with soup. Pour into casserole and bake at 350° for 45 to 60 minutes. 6-8 servings.

3/4 cup = C-15; P-21; F-6

Exchange: 2 meat, 1 bread

SPANISH RICE WITH MEAT

```
1 medium onion, chopped ..................... 100 grams
1 large green pepper, chopped ................. 100 grams
2 tsp. butter or margarine...................... 10 grams
Approx. 12½ ozs. ground round (raw) ............ 370 grams
1 cup instant rice — dry wt. .................... 130 grams
1-1/3 cup water
1/2 tsp. salt
1-2/3 cups tomato sauce........................ 400 grams
5 large ripe olives, sliced ....................... 50 grams
```

Season to taste with salt, pepper, Worchestershire Sauce and Tabasco Sauce.
Saute onion and green pepper in butter. Add tomato sauce, olives and seasonings. Brown meat and add to mixture. Cook rice in salted water according to directions on package. When tender, add to meat mixture.

Turn into a casserole and bake in a 325° oven for 1/2 hour. If mixture becomes too dry, add a small amount of water.
Yield: 6 servings.

1/6 recipe = C-26; P-22; F-9

Exchange: 1½ bread; 1 B vegetable; 1½ meat; and 1 fat

CHILI

```
1 (16 oz.) can tomatoes
1 lb. very lean ground beef
1 (16 oz.) can kidney beans
    and liquid
1 large onion
2 cloves garlic, minced ............................. free
chili powder, salt & pepper (to taste) .................. free
```

Brown hamburger and onion. Add salt, pepper, garlic, chili powder and tomatoes. Stir and simmer. Put kidney beans in blender and whirl until soupy. Add beans, simmer for 1/2 to 1 hr. and serve.

Total recipe = C-87; P-165; F-45
1/4 recipe = C-22; P-41; F-11
1/6 recipe = C-15; P-28; F-8

Exchange: 1/4 recipe = 1 bread, 1 Veg. B, 3½ meat
1/6 recipe = 1 bread, 3 meat

LASAGNA

5 oz. ground round, lean and cooked . . . . 140 grams
1/2 cup tomato sauce . . . . 120 grams
Scant 1/2 cup tomato juice . . . . 100 grams
1 tbsp. onion, finely chopped . . . . 15 grams
1 oz. American cheese . . . . 20 grams
1/2 cup + 2 tbsp. cottage cheese . . . . 100 grams
1 tsp. spaghetti sauce mix . . . . 5 grams
Seasonings as desired (salt, oregano, garlic)
2 cups lasanga-type noodles, dry wt. . . . . 120 grams

Cook noodles in salted water until tender. Sear meat in a skillet until brown. Remove from skillet. To same skillet, add tomato sauce, tomato juice, onion, American cheese and cottage cheese. Stir and cook until well blended. Add seasonings and simmer slowly for 10 minutes. Mix sauce and noodles together very gently. Place mixture in a baking dish and bake in a 350° oven for 30 minutes. If mixture seems dry, add a small amount of water.

Yield: 4 servings.

1 serving (1/4 of recipe) = C-26; P-20; F-8.

Exchange: 1/2 milk; 1 bread; 1 B. vegetable; 1 meat; 1 fat.

QUICK FILLET OF SOLE

1/2 lb. fillet of sole
1 can cream of shrimp soup
1 4 oz. can shrimp pieces
1½ cups dry quick cooking rice

Wash fish, lay in baking dish, pour soup and shrimp over top. Bake at 325° for 1/2 hour. While baking, prepare rice. Serve over rice.

Total recipe = C-60; P-98; F-21
1/3 recipe = C-20; P-33; F-7
1/4 recipe = C-15; P-25; F-5

Exchange: 1/3 recipe = 1 soup, 1/2 bread, 3 meat, *add 1 fat
1/4 recipe = 1 bread, 2½ meat

CABBAGE ROLLS

10 to 12 cabbage leaves
1 lb. very lean ground beef
1 cup quick-cooking rice, raw
1 small onion, chopped
1/2 tsp. salt
1 16 oz. can tomatoes
5-10 mushrooms, sliced

Pull off cabbage leaves. Rinse in cold water. Place leaves in 2 cups boiling water to soften. Cover pan and turn off heat to let leaves steam while preparing stuffing.

Prepare stuffing by mixing ground beef, rice, chopped onion, and salt in mixing bowl. Carefully remove cabbage leaves from pot.

Place a heaping tbsp. of mixture in the center of each leaf. Fold meat in the leaf envelope style. Secure rolled leaf with toothpick.

Place each roll, fold side down, in pan. Pour tomatoes and mushrooms over the top. Cover with lid, bake at 350° for about 1 hour or until cabbage rolls are firm.

Total recipe = C-123; P-144; F-45
1/4 recipe = C-31; P-36; F-11
1/6 recipe = C-21; P-24; F-8
1/8 recipe = C-15; P-18; F-6

Exchange: 1/4 recipe = 1½ bread, 1 veg. B, 3 meat and 1/2 fat.
1/6 recipe = 1 bread, 1 veg. B, 2 meat
1/8 recipe = 1/2 bread, 1 veg. B, 1½ meat

SAUCES

HOLLANDAISE SAUCE

4 tsp. butter (melted) . . . . 20 grams
1 egg yolk . . . . 20 grams
1 tbsp. lemon juice . . . . 15 grams
1/2 tsp. salt

Blend, warm and serve.

Total recipe = C-0; P-3; F-22
1/2 recipe = C-0; P-2; F-11

Exchange: 2 fat

BENIHANA GINGER SAUCE

1/4 cup chopped fresh ginger
1 cup chopped onion .... 160 grams
3 strips lemon peel .... free
1/2 cup vinegar .... free
1 tsp. monosodium glutamate (msg) .... free
1 pint soy sauce
From 1/4 lemon — lemon juice .... free

Whirl ginger, onion, lemon peel, vinegar, and msg. in blender for about 1 minute. Add soy sauce and lemon juice and mix thoroughly.

Serve with Teppanyaki (beef, seafood, poultry, and vegetables, sauteed Japanese style in a little oil on a hot grill) or as a meat and vegetable sauce.

Total recipe = C-64; P-29; F-5
1 tbsp. = C-1; P-1; F-0
Or
1 free exchange

WHITE SAUCE

1 cup 2% milk
4 tsp. flour
1 tbsp. butter
1 tsp. Worcestershire sauce .... free
Dash cayenne pepper .... free
Salt to taste .... free

Blend last 5 ingredients over medium heat, then add milk, stirring constantly. Heat thoroughly and serve.

Total recipe = C-20; P-8; F-17
1/3 recipe = C-6; P-3; F-6
1/5 recipe = C-4; P-2; F-3
1/6 recipe = C-3; P-1; F-3

Exchange: 1/3 recipe = 1/2 milk
and 1/2 fat
1/5 recipe = 1/3 milk
and 1/2 fat
1/6 recipe = 1/4 milk
and 1/2 fat

TARTAR SAUCE = 1/3 cup

2 tbsp. mayonnaise . . . . 30 grams
1/4 tsp. capers, chopped . . . . free
1 green onion, chopped . . . . 5 grams
1/2 tsp. dill pickle, chopped . . . . free
1/3 tsp. parsley, chopped . . . . free

Combine, let set in refrigerator and serve.

Total recipe = C-0; P-0; F-26

Exchange: 1 Recipe = 5 fat
1/2 recipe = 2½ fat
1/3 recipe = 1½ fat

BREADS and BREAKFAST HELPS

COTTAGE CHEESE PANCAKES

3 eggs . . . . 150 grams
1/3 cup + 1 tbsp. flour . . . . 40 grams
1/4 tsp. salt
2/3 cup cottage cheese . . . . 150 grams

Separate eggs. Beat whites until stiff and yolks until lemon colored. To yolks add flour, salt and cottage cheese. When thoroughly mixed, fold in egg whites. This makes a very light pancake and if the griddle is smooth, no grease is necessary.
Yield: 6 large cakes

Total recipe = C-35; P-43; F-24
Each cake = C-6; P-7; F-4

Exchange: 1/2 milk and 1 meat

BANANA BREAD

*1/2 cup sugar .... 100 grams
1/2 cup butter or shortening .... 114 grams
2 eggs .... 100 grams
3 small or 2 lg. mashed bananas .... 300 grams
1¾ cups flour .... 230 grams
Pinch of salt .... free
1 tsp. soda .... free
1/2 tsp. baking powder .... free

Makes approximately 16 slices.
Bake at 350° for 50-55 minutes.

Total recipe = C-339; P-40; F-106
Each slice = C-21; P-3; F-7

Exchange: 1 bread, 1/2 fruit and
1 fat

CARROT BREAD

*1/2 cup sugar .... 100 grams
1/2 cup butter or shortening .... 114 grams
2 eggs .... 100 grams
1¾ cups mashed carrots .... 300 grams
1¾ cups flour .... 230 grams
Pinch of salt .... free
1 tsp. soda .... free
1/2 tsp. baking powder .... free
1/4 tsp. ginger .... free
1/2 tsp. cinnamon .... free

Makes approximately 16 slices.
See directions below. Bake at
350° for 50-55 minutes.

Total recipe = C-291; P-46; F-106
Each slice = C-19; P-3; F-7

Exchange: 1 bread, 1/2 veg. B
and 1 fat

DIRECTIONS FOR BOTH RECIPES:
Mix in order given: cream butter and sugar together, add eggs &
bananas (or carrots) and mix thoroughly. Sift dry ingredients together,
add to mixture and mix thoroughly. Pour into loaf pan and bake.

*Note: The sugar in these two recipes is figured into the total value. The
amount of sugar versus the amount of flour is acceptable in this
instance.

BAKED APPLE FOR BREAKFAST

1 small baked cinnamon apple
1/4 cup cottage cheese
1/2 cup skim milk
Dash vanilla . . . . free
Sugar substitute = to 1 or 1½ tsp. sugar . . . . free
2 crushed graham crackers

Fill center of apple with cottage cheese. Add vanilla and sugar substitute to milk and pour over apple. Sprinkle with graham cracker crumbs. Can serve warm or cold.

Total recipe = C-28; P-14; F-4

Exchange: 1 fruit, 3/4 bread, 1/2 milk, 1 meat.

JAM

RASPBERRY JAM*

1/4 tsp. ascorbic acid
3 cups raspberries
1½ tbsp. liquid sweetener
1½ tbsp. cold water
1½ tsp. unflavored gelatin
Red food coloring

Soften gelatin in cold water. Combine berries and sweetener in saucepan. Place over high heat. Stir constantly until mixture comes to a boil. Remove from heat. Add softened gelatin, return to heat and continue to cook for 1 minute. Remove from heat, and add ascorbic acid powder and red food coloring. Poor into clean half-pint jars and seal.

Refrigerate or freeze. Makes 2 half-pint jars. 1 tbsp. = 5 calories; 1 gm. Carbo., trace of protein and trace of fat. If only 1 tbsp. is used, it need not be calculated in the diet.

Exchange: 4 tbsp. = 1/2 fruit

*May use other berries if desired

COOKIES and CANDY

FUDGE

1 square unsweetened chocolate
1 cup evaporated milk
2 tsp. vanilla
1 tsp. liquid sweetener
1 pkg. vanilla or chocolate diet pudding mix

Melt chocolate in top of double boiler, over boiling water. Add evaporated milk and mix well. Cook for 2-3 minutes. Add vanilla and sweetener. Spread on small foil pan and chill. Cut in 8 pieces. Candy may be served plain or formed into balls and rolled in pudding powder or nuts.

Total recipe = C-15; P-0; F-20

Exchange: 1 recipe = 1½ fruit and 4 fat
1 piece rolled in pudding powder = 1/2 fat. Rolled in nuts = 1 fat.

COOKIE'S BROWNIES

2 squares unsweetened baking chocolate
3 tbsp. liquid sweetener
2 cups cake flour
1½ cups chopped walnuts
2 eggs
2/3 cup butter
4 tsp. vanilla
1 tsp. salt
1 tsp. soda

Melt chocolate and butter in double boiler top. Cool slightly. Add sweetener, vanilla and dry ingredients. Bake at 325° for 20 minutes. Makes 62 brownies.

Each brownie = C-3; P-1; F-5

Exchange: 1 brownie = 1/5 bread + 1 fat
Five brownies = 1 bread + 5 fat

──────── CHOCOLATE CHIP COOKIES ────────

1 cup sifted flour
1/2 tsp. baking soda
1/4 tsp. salt
1/2 cup butter
4 tsp. liquid sweetener
1/2 tsp. vanilla
1 egg, beaten
1/2 cup semi-sweet chocolate chips

Sift dry ingredients together. Cream butter, add sweetener, vanilla and egg. Blend well. Add flour mixture and beat well. Stir in chocolate chips. Drop by teaspoonful onto lightly greased baking sheet. Bake 8-10 minutes. Makes 36 cookies.

Each cookie = C-3.5; P-0.5; F-3.5

Exchange: 4 cookies = 1 bread and 3 fat

──────── CINNAMON SPICE COOKIES ────────

5 tbsp. butter
1 cup flour
1/2 tsp. baking powder
Pinch of salt
2 tsp. liquid sweetener
1 tsp. vanilla
1 tbsp. milk or coffee
1 tsp. cinnamon

Cream butter until light and fluffy. Blend in flour, baking powder, cinnamon and salt. Mix sweetener with vanilla, and milk or coffee. Stir into flour mixture and mix thoroughly. Shape dough into 30 even-sized balls and place on cookie sheet. Flatten balls with a fork dipped in cold water. Bake 10-15 minutes at 375°.

4 cookies = C-10; P-0; F-5

Exchange: 4 cookies = 1/2 Bread and 1 fat

PEANUT BUTTER COOKIES

1/4 cup butter
1/2 cup peanut butter
2 tbsp. liquid sweetener
1 tsp. baking powder
1/4 tsp. salt
1/3 cup milk
1 egg
1 tsp. vanilla
1 cup flour

Cream butter, peanut butter and sweetener. Sift dry ingredients together, and add alternately with milk, egg and vanilla. Make into 48 cookies. Bake at 375° for 10 minutes.

Each cookie = C-2.5; P-1; F-2.5

Exchange: 5 cookies = 1 bread and 2 fat and 1/2 meat

OATMEAL COOKIES

1/2 cup margarine
1 egg
1 tsp. liquid sweetener
1/4 cup milk
1 cup sifted flour
1/8 tsp. baking soda
1 tsp. cinnamon
1/2 tsp. nutmeg
1/4 tsp. salt
1 tsp. vanilla
1/2 cup raisins
1 cup rolled oats

Cream margarine, add beaten egg, sweetener and milk. Sift and mix dry ingredients. Add them to first creamed mixture. Beat in vanilla, raisins and rolled oats. Drop by teaspoon onto greased cookie sheet and bake at 375° for 15 minutes. Makes 30 cookies.

One cookie = C-7; P-1; F-4

Exchange: Two cookies = 1 bread and 1½ fat

GRANOLA

3 tbsp. honey
2 tbsp. oil
1/2 tsp. vanilla
6 tbsp. wheat germ
1½ cups rolled oats
1/2 cup coconut
6 tbsp. soy beans
6 tbsp. pecans
1/2 cup sesame seeds

Mix together and bake on oiled cookie sheet for 20-30 minutes at 300°. Stir every 2 to 3 minutes, so mixture browns evenly.

1/3 cup = C-15; P-5; F-10

Exchange: 1/3 cup = 1 bread, 2 fat

LIZ' HOMEMADE GRANOLA

Old-fashioned rolled oats .... 100 grams
Old-fashioned wheat flakes .... 100 grams
Shredded unsweetened coconut .... 100 grams
Sunflower seeds .... 100 grams
Brown sugar .... 100 grams
3 tbsp. Salad oil
2 tbsp. water

Mix all ingredients thoroughly. Spread on a cookie sheet. Bake at 225° for one hour. If you press it together a bit it will stick together while baking and you may break it into cookie-like pieces. If you want it crumbly, stir it a couple of times while baking.

This is great for backpacking. It makes approximately 400 grams.

100 grams = C-70; P-14; F-42
20 grams = C-14; P-3; F-8

Exchange: 20 grams = 1 bread & 2 fat

DESSERTS

DIET CUSTARD FOR 2

Scant 3/4 cup skim milk . . . . 172 grams
1 egg, beaten
3/4 to 1 tsp. vanilla
1/2 tsp. liquid sweetener
Dash salt
Dash mace

Combine first 5 ingredients. Divide into two custard cups. Sprinkle custard with mace. Place in hot water and bake at 350° until knife inserted in center comes out clean.

Each serving = C-5; P-5; F-3

Exchange: 1/2 whole milk

BANANA CUSTARD

Add 50 grams (1/2 small) banana, sliced, to plain custard recipe.

1/2 recipe = C-11; P-6; F-7

Exchange: 1/2 milk and 1/2 fruit

PINEAPPLE FLUFF

1 pkg. lemon or lime diet jello
1 large can diet crushed pineapple, drained
1 pkg. whipped topping mix

Dissolve jello in 1½ cups boiling water. Add 3/4 cup fruit juice and stir. Let thicken. Stir in 2 cups of whipped topping and pineapple. Put in refrigerator to set. Makes 6 servings.

1 serving = C-10; P-0; F-0

Exchange: 1 serving = 1 fruit

TOPPING DELIGHT

1 cup applesauce .... 200 grams
1 pkg. prepared whipped topping (2 cups)
1/4 tsp. cinnamon .... free

Makes twelve 1/4 cup servings.
Mix and serve.

Total recipe = C-26; P-4; F-16
1/4 cup = C-2; P-1; F-4

Exchange: 1 fat

ORANGE PINEAPPLE SHERBET

1 6 oz. can frozen unsweetened orange juice concentrate
1 6 oz. can frozen unsweetened pineapple juice concentrate
3½ cups cold water
2 tbsp. liquid sweetener
1 cup non-fat dry milk

Set refrigerator at coldest setting. Put all ingredients into a 2 qt. bowl in order listed above. Beat enough to blend. Pour into ice cube trays; freeze 1 to 2 hours until partly frozen. Remove to larger chilled mixer bowl. Beat on low speed until mixture softens, then beat on high speed 3 to 5 minutes until creamy but not liquid. Freeze in freezer containers. 1/2 cup = 58 calories.

1/2 cup = C-13; P-0; F-0

Exchange: 1/4 cup skim milk and 1 fruit

APPLE GRAHAM CRISP

83 grams apple slices, w.p. (1 medium apple)
Liquid sweetener to taste
Cinnamon to taste

Put in individual serving dish. Crush 1 graham cracker — add 1 tsp. butter. Sprinkle over top of apple slices.
Bake at 350° until bubbly.
Makes 1 serving.

Total recipe = C-14; P-1; F-5

Exchange: 1 fruit, 1 fat, 1/4 bread

SPICE PUMPKIN PIE

1/2 cup pumpkin .... 100 grams
1/2 egg
1/4 cup milk .... 60 grams
1 tsp. melted butter .... 6 grams
Salt, cinnamon, nutmeg, ginger and cloves to taste

Beat the whole egg and measure out half for the recipe.
Combine all ingredients and pour into unbaked shell. Bake at 350° until knife inserted slightly off-center comes out clean.

1/2 pie = C-16; P-5; F-11

Exchange: 1 B vegetable; 1/2 bread; 2 fat

ONE CRUST INDIVIDUAL PIE

1/3 cup flour .... 30 grams
1 tbsp. solid shortening .... 12 grams
1/8 tsp. salt
1 tbsp. water

Follow the usual procedure for making pie crust.
Use an individual pie pan measuring 5 inches across the top.

Total recipe = C-23; P-3; F-12

Exchange: 1½ bread; 2 fat

APPLESAUCE*

1 lb. cooking apples
1 (12 oz.) can Diet Shasta Red Apple .... free
1/4 tsp. artificial sweetener (to taste) .... free
1/2 tsp. cinnamon .... free
4 thin lemon slices (optional) .... free

Rinse, core, peel and cut apples in lengths. Combine all ingredients in large skillet. Simmer until apples are tender, about 10 minutes. Cool and chill. Makes 2½ cups.

Total recipe = C-55; P-0; F-0
1/3 recipe = C-18; P-0; F-0
1/5 recipe = C-11; P-0; F-0
(1/2 cup)

Exchange: 1/3 recipe = 2 fruit
1/5 recipe (1/2 cup) = 1 fruit

STRAWBERRY-MELON DESSERT*

2 tsp. unflavored gelatin	free
1 (12 oz.) can Diet Shasta Strawberry	free
1/2 tsp. artificial liquid sweetener	free
1/4 tsp. strawberry extract	free
Dash salt	free
2 tsp. lemon juice	free
1½ cups whole or sliced strawberries	
1 small cantaloupe	

Sprinkle gelatin over 1/2 cup Diet Shasta, stirring until dissolved. Heat. Add remaining Diet Shasta, sweetener, extract, salt and lemon juice. Cool, then chill until mixture begins to jell. Fold in berries. Remove rind and seeds and cut cantaloupe in 1/2 inch slices. Spoon sauce over melon slices. Makes 5 or 6 servings.

Total recipe = C-49; P-0; F-0
1/5 recipe = C-10; P-0; F-0
1/6 recipe = C-8; P-0; F-0

Exchange: 1/5 recipe = 1 fruit
1/6 recipe = 1 fruit

*Used by permission of Shasta Beverage Co.

Part 7

RESOURCE LISTS
GLOSSARY
ALPHABETICAL INDEX

Appendix

HANDBOOKS AND PAMPHLETS

These are particularly useful for those with diabetes:

American Diabetes Association. Forecast. 1 West 48th Street, New York, N.Y. 10020. A magazine published every other month.

Ames Company. Diabetes in the News, 3553 W. Peterson Ave., Chicago, Illinois 60659. A free newspaper.

Behrman, M., A cookbook for Diabetics. New York, American Diabetes Association, 1959.

Bennett, Margaret. The Peripatetic Diabetic, Hawthorn Books, Inc., New York, 1969.

Boshell, Buris R., The Diabetic at Work and Play, Charles C. Thomas, Springfield, Illinois, 1973.

Composition of Foods. Agriculture Handbook No. 8, Superintendent of Documents, U.S. Government Printing Office, Washington D.C. 20402.

Diabetes. Public Health Service, Pub. No. 137. Washington, D.C., U.S. Government Printing Office, 1968.

Dolger, H., and Seeman, B. How to Live with Diabetes. New York, Pyramid Books, Inc., 1958. Rev. Ed., 1966.

Duncan, G. A. Modern Pilgrim's Progress for Diabetes, 2nd ed. Philadelphia, W. B. Saunders Co., 1967.

Etzwiler, D. D., and Robb, J. R. First International Workshop on Diabetes and Camping.

Feet First. U.S. Dept. of Health, Education and Welfare. Supt. of Documents; U.S. Government Printing Office; Washington, D.C., 1970.

Gibbons, Euell, and Gibbons, Joe. Feast on a Diabetic Diet. David McKay Company, Inc. New York, 1969.

Graber, et al. Diabetes and Pregnancy, Vanderbilt University Press, Nashville, Tennessee, 1973.

Joslin Clinic. Diabetic Manual, 11th Edition, Lea and Febiger, Philadelphia, 1973.

Rogue Valley Memorial Hospital. Delectable Dining for Diabetics, Medford, Oregon, 1969.

Rosenthal, Helen, and Rosenthal, Joseph. Diabetic Care in Pictures, 4th Ed., Philadelphia, Lippencott, 1968.

Schmitt, George F. Diabetes for Diabetics, Diabetes Press of America, Miami, Florida, 1965.

Stephens, J. W. et al. A Diabetic Diary, Portland, Oregon. Revised 1972.

Stephens, J. W., Page, O. C., and Hare, R. L. Diet Handbook for Diabetics, Portland, Oregon, Rev. Ed., 1975.

Strachan, Clarice. The Diabetics Cookbook, University of Texas Press, Medical Arts Publishing Foundation, 1972.

University of Oregon Medical School and Hospitals. Handbook of Diabetes Management, Rev. Ed., 1974.

Vanderpoel, Sally. The Care and Feeding of Your Diabetic Child, Frederick Fell, Inc., New York, 1968.

These are particularly useful for the professional:

Burke, Elizabeth, R. N., *Insulin Injection; The Site and The Technique.* A. J. N., December 1972.

Burke, Elizabeth, R. N., *Training Program in Diabetes Care.* Nursing Outlook, August 1971.

Diabetes Mellitus. Eli Lilly Company, Indianapolis, Indiana 46205, 1973. (2nd edition, second revision).

Derr, Susan, R. N., M. S., *Testing for Glycosuria.* A. J. N., July 1970.

Education and Management of the Patient With Diabetes Mellitus. Ames Co., Elkhart, Indiana, 1973.

Guthrie, Diana, R. N. and Guthrie, Richard, M. D., *Coping With Diabetic Keto- acidosis.* Nursing '73, November.

Guthrie, Diana, R. N., M. S. P. H., *Diabetic Children.* Nursing '73, March.

Jordan, Judith, R. N., and Shipp, Joseph, M. D., *The Primary Health Care Pro- fessional Was A Nurse,* A. J. N., May 1971.

Krosnic, Arthur, M. D., *The Nurse and Diabetes Control.* The New Jersey State Department of Health, Trenton, N.J.

Stephens, J. W., Page, O. C., Hare, R. L., Drake, R., *Treatment of Juvenile Diabe- tes Mellitus.* Ped. Digest 9:45, 1967.

Special Report. Principles of Nutrition and Dietary Recommendations for Patients with Diabetes Mellitus: 1971. *Diabetes,* September, 1971.

RESOURCE LIST FOR ADDITIONAL INFORMATION, MATERIALS, AND SERVICES

American Diabetes Association, Inc.
1 West 48th Street
New York, N.Y. 10020

American Diabetes Association
Oregon Affiliate
P.O. Box 13510
Portland, Oregon 97213

American Foundation for the Blind, Inc.
15 West 16th St.
New York, N.Y. 10011
Products for the blind. Send for catalogue: Aids and Appliances

Diabetes Association of Greater Cleveland
2022 Lee
Cleveland, Ohio 44118
Instant Glucose: Write for current order form

Blind Commission for the State of Oregon
535 S.E. 12th
Portland, Oregon 97214

Diabetes Treatment and Education Center
Good Samaritan Hospital & Medical Center
Portland, Oregon 97210

Write for identification tag forms.
   W. A. Morrow Co., Inc.
   8115 S.E. 28th St., P.O. Box 188
   Mercer Island, Washington 98040

   Medic Alert Foundation
   P.O. Box 1009
   Turlock, California 95380

Filmstrips on Urine Testing; one for mild, adult onset, one for juvenile onset. Available from Pacific Productions, P.O. Box 625, Beaverton, Oregon 97005.

Filmstrip on Insulin Injection Technique available: Pacific Productions, P.O. Box 625, Beaverton, Oregon 97005.

GLOSSARY OF TERMS

ACETEST: a method for determining the amount of acetone present in the urine.

ACETOHEXAMIDE: (the chemical name for Dymelor) a Sulfonylurea medication useful in controlling maturity onset diabetes.

ACETONE: an end product of fat metabolism, most commonly found in the urine when diabetes is out of control, after lengthy fasting or exercise.

ACIDOSIS: see Ketoacidosis.

ADIPOSE FAT: serves as a fuel reserve or energy source for the body. When excessive in amount it causes one to appear obese. It is composed mainly of triglyceride which the body derives from ingested carbohydrate and fat.

ADULT ONSET DIABETES: (maturity onset diabetes) the mild type of diabetes that occurs most commonly after forty years of age; frequently associated with being overweight. This form of diabetes is rarely associated with ketoacidosis, as insulin production and secretion still occur, though in a less efficient manner.

"AIR HUNGER": See Kussmaul breathing.

ALPHA CELL: one of the types of cells found within the Islets of Langerhans, responsible for the production and secretion of glucagon.

ARTERIOSLEROSIS: (hardening of the arteries) refers to thickening, hardening, and loss of elasticity of the blood vessels. It occurs more frequently and at an earlier age in diabetics.

ATHLETE'S FOOT: a fungus infection of the foot.

BENEDICT'S TEST: an older method for determining the presence of sugar in the urine.

BETA CELL: a type of cell found within the Islets of Langerhans in the pancreas, responsible for the production and secretion of insulin.

BIGUANIDES: a group of drugs effective in lowering the blood sugar in the adult onset diabetic. These drugs act in some way to improve the cellular intake of glucose.

CALORIE: amount of heat required to raise 1 gm. of water 1 degree centigrade; measurement of food energy.

CARBOHYDRATE: the chemical elements of some foods which include sugars and starches. They are necessary for body energy. These are foods that grow from the ground. Milk also contains carbohydrate.

CATARACT: a clouding of the lens of the eye.

CHLORPROPAMIDE: (the chemical name for Diabinese) a Sulfonylurea medication useful in controlling maturity onset diabetes.

CLINISTIX: a simple method for determining the presence of sugar in the urine. (This method is not usually suggested for the patient requiring insulin.)

CLINITEST: a method for determining the presence and amount of sugar in the urine. (This is the suggested method for the patient requiring insulin.)

CRYSTALLINE INSULIN: see Regular insulin.

CYCLAMATE: a chemical which renders a sweet taste and has no calories.

DBI-TD: (Phenformin) a biguanide preparation. It is useful in the control of maturity onset diabetes.

DIABINESE: (Chlorpropamide) a Sulfonylurea medication useful in controlling maturity onset diabetes.

DIABETES MELLITUS: a generalized metabolic disorder associated with higher than normal blood sugar levels and sometimes the presence of sugar in the urine. Results from inadequate production or utilization of insulin.

DIABETIC COMA: a complication of untreated ketoacidosis.

DIABETIC NEURITIS: one of the complications of diabetes, involving the nerve endings. It sometimes manifests itself as pain, sometimes as decreased sensation to the affective area, particularly the feet and legs.

DIASTIX: a method for determining the presence of sugar in the urine.

DIET PLAN: a plan of eating. In diabetes, diet planning should restrict sugar and contain the same amount of carbohydrate, protein and fat each day. Meals should be eaten on schedule and good nutrition observed.

DIETETIC: referring to foods which have been specially prepared for people who have problems with nutrition. *Does not mean diabetic*, although some dietetic foods may be specially prepared for the diabetic.

DIGESTION: food being changed into a form which the body can use.

DYMELOR: (Acetohexamide) a Sulfonylurea medication useful in controlling maturity onset diabetes.

FASTING BLOOD GLUCOSE: blood sugar drawn following a period of 6 to 10 hours without eating. Normal is 60 to 110 mg.%.

FAT: element found in many foods. Fat is necessary to absorb certain vitamins, for digestive purposes, energy and storage. Fat yields nine calories per gram.

FEBRILE: having fever.

GLAUCOMA: a disease of the eye, characterized by increased pressure within the chamber of the eye.

GLUCAGON: a hormone produced in the alpha cell of the Islet of Langerhans which raises the blood sugar level.

GLUCOSE: a form of sugar.

GLUCOSE TOLERANCE TEST: a method of diagnosing diabetes mellitus. Blood and urine samples are obtained at prescribed intervals following the ingestion of a concentrated glucose drink.

GLYCEMIA: the presence of glucose in the blood.

GLYCOSURIA: (glucosuria) the presence of glucose in the urine.

GRAM: a unit of weight in the metric system. The gram scale is useful for weighing prescribed amounts of food.

HARDENING OF THE ARTERIES: see Arteriosclerosis.

HEREDITY: the development of traits and characteristics possessed and passed by one generation to another.

HUB: the part of the needle which fits onto the syringe.

HYPERGLYCEMIA: high blood sugar — above acceptable levels.

HYPOGLYCEMIA: low blood sugar — below acceptable levels.

IMPOTENCE: inability to be sexually active.

INJECTION: method of putting insulin into body tissue through a needle; "shot".

INSULIN: a hormone, normally produced by the beta cell in the Islet of Langerhans in the pancreas, which lowers the blood sugar.

INSULIN REACTION: see Hypoglycemia. A set of symptoms produced when the blood sugar reaches a low level. Symptoms may include shakiness, perspiration, nervousness, tingling around the lips, behavior changes, etc.

ISLETS OF LANGERHANS: clusters of cells in the pancreas; responsible for the production of insulin and glucagon.

ISOPHANE INSULIN: see NPH insulin.

JUVENILE ONSET DIABETES: (growth onset diabetes) the type of diabetes that occurs most commonly in young people. The symptoms of increasing thirst and frequency of urination are the result of a deficiency of insulin.

KETOACIDOSIS: a complication of uncontrolled diabetes resulting from lack of insulin and associated with an accumulation of ketones in the blood (and urine). Other signs of uncontrolled diabetes are elevation of the blood glucose (with 2 percent or more glucose in the urine) and dehydration.

KETONE BODIES: by-products of fat metabolism found in the urine.

KETOSTIX: a method of detecting ketones in the urine.

KUSSMAUL BREATHING: ("air hunger") an increased rate of breathing commonly associated with acidosis.

LENTE INSULIN: an intermediate-acting insulin which begins its action two hours after injection, reaches a peak of action at 8-12 hours, and is over in 20-24 hours.

MANNITOL: a sweet-tasting starch found in many dietetic foods. Calories must be counted.

METABOLISM: the physical and chemical changes involved in the utilization of food.

NEEDLE: the long shaft attached to the syringe through which insulin is injected into body tissues.

NEPHROPATHY: disease of the kidney.

NEURITIS: inflammation of a nerve or nerves.

NEUROPATHY: any disease of the nerves.

NORMAL BLOOD SUGAR: acceptable levels of blood sugar in relation to the last meal. Fasting = 60-120 mg./100 ml.; 1 hour after a meal = 100-160 mg./100 ml. Correct for plasma determination.

NPH INSULIN: an intermediate-acting insulin which begins acting two hours after injection, reaches a peak of action at 8-12 hours and is over in 20-24 hours.

OBESITY: abnormal amount of fat in the body. The term is generally used when body weight is 20% over that which is considered normal for the individual.

OPTHALMOLOGIST: a physician who specializes in the treatment of disorders of the eye.

ORINASE: (Tolbutamide) a Sulfonylurea medication useful in controlling maturity onset diabetes.

PANCREAS: a gland lying behind the stomach; responsible for the production of hormones, insulin and glucagon.

PHENFORMIN: (a biguanide, DBI-TD) useful in controlling maturity onset diabetes.

PODIATRIST: a person specially trained in the diagnosis and treatment of foot disorders.

POLYDYPSIA: excessive thirst.

POLYPHASIA: excessive hunger.

POLYURIA: excessive secretion of urine.

POST-PRANDIAL: following a meal.

PROTEIN: a complex food containing amino acids. It is necessary for growth and repair of body tissue. Present in meat, fish, and dairy products.

REGULAR INSULIN: (crystalline insulin) a rapidly acting insulin which begins acting 30 minutes after injection, reaches its peak in 3-4 hours, and is finished acting at 6-8 hours.

RENAL THRESHOLD: the point at which the kidneys allow glucose to escape into the urine.

RETINOPATHY: disorder of the retina of the eye.

SACCHARIN: a chemical which renders a sweet taste and has no calories.

SEMI-LENTE INSULIN: a variation of Lente insulin with a beginning action about 1 hour after injection, a peak of 6-8 hours, and a duration of 10-12 hours.

SOMATOSTATIN: inhibitor of secretion of several hormones (e.g., growth hormone, insulin, glucagon).

SORBITOL: a sweet-tasting starch found in many dietetic foods. Calories must be counted.

SPILLING POINT: see Renal Threshold.

STARCH: a complex carbohydrate which is slowly metabolized. Starches are in foods which grow from the ground and rarely have a sweet taste.

SUCROSE: readily available or simple carbohydrate; another name for table sugar.

SUGAR: a rapidly used carbohydrate. Sugars are in foods which grow from the gound and usually have a sweet taste. Examples are dextrose, fructose. Sugar in milk is lactose. Sugar in the bloodstream is glucose.

SULFONYLUREAS: a group of medications which stimulate the pancreas to secrete insulin.

SYRINGE: the device which holds a measured amount of insulin for injection.

TESTAPE: a method for testing urine for glucose.

TOLBUTAMIDE: see Orinase.

TOLINASE: (Tolazamide) a Sulfonylurea medication useful in controlling maturity onset diabetes.

TRIGLYCERIDE: a lipid compound composed of glycerol and fatty acids.

ULTRA-LENTE INSULIN: a long-acting insulin.

VITRECTOMY: surgery of the eye to remove vitreous.

VITREOUS: fluid in the eyeball.

Index

A

Acetest—urine test for ketones, 112
Acetohexamide—(see Dymelor), 82-83
  100
Acetone, 112, 125
  in blood, 125
  in diabetic acidosis, 125
  in urine, 112
  tests for, 112
  when to test for, 112, 125
Acidosis—(see diabetic keto-
  acidosis), 124-125
Acute illness, 25, 115-120
  Routines for management, 115-120
    Adjustment of insulin during, 116
    Illness with fever, 116-120
    Liquid diets, 116
    Stomach Flu, 115
Adult onset d.m., 17-26
  Acute illness, 25, 115
  Blood glucose responses (graph), 18
  Characteristics, 18
  Complications, 19
  Control, 20-23
  Diet—(see treatment), 21
  Employment, 20, 143
  Exercise, 21-22
  F.D.A. warning, 23, 82
Health hazards, 19
  Obesity, 19
  Other, 20
  Employability, 20, 143
  Insulin (see treatment), 21
  Obesity, 19, 134-137
  Objectives of treatment, 20-21
  Plasma insulin responses (graph), 18
  Reasons to treat, 19-20
  Symptoms of, 17
  Treatment, 19, 21-25
    Diet: type, 21
    Evaluation of treatment, 23-24
    Exercise, 21
    Illness—treatment during, 24-25
    Insulin, 21, 23, 84-100
    Oral tablets, 21, 23, 82-83

Air hunger (see Kussmaul respirations),
  125
Alcohol, 78-79
  Caloric values, 78
  Effect on diabetes, 78-79
Alpha cell and glucagon, 13-14
Appendix, 180
Argon Laser, 130
Arteriosclerosis (see atherosclerosis),
  79, 127
Atherosclerosis, 127
  Dietary fat and, 79-80
Artificial Sweeteners, 45
Athlete's foot, 122

B

Berson, Dr. Solomon, 18
Beta cells, 13
Bibliography, 180
Biguanides—DBI, 82
Blood glucose, 8-9
  Control of in non-diabetic, 8
  Normal levels, 9
  Source, 8
Blue Cross, hospital insurance, 144
Body weight—ideal, 134

C

Calloses—care of, 122
Calorie, 22, 46
Camps, summer for children, 33
Carbohydrate, 38, 46
Cataracts, 129
Cereal, food value, 53 70
Chlorpropamide—(see Diabinese),
  23, 82, 100
Clinistix—urine test for glucose, 108, 110
Clinitest—urine test for glucose, 108-111
Coma, 107, 124
Complications, 124-131
  Associated with adult onset
    diabetes, 19-20
  atherosclerosis, 127
  disorders of vision, 128-131
  Ketoacidosis, 124-125

Nephropathy, 128
Neuritis, 126
Contraceptives—use of, 139-141
Corns—care of, 122
Craighead, Dr. J.E., 13
Crystalline insulin, 87
Cyclamate, 44

D

Dairy products, food value, 57, 58, 61, 73, 74
DBI-TD, 82
Diabetes Mellitus
   Adult—onset, 17
   Airmen Medical Certification, 148
   Causes—see inheritance, 10, 11, 12
      Lesions of pancreas, 15
   Definition, 8
   Development of, 10
   Diet in, 21, 36-45, 46-66, 67
   Hypoglycemia in, 13, 83, 100-107
   Incidence, 14
   Indications for testing for, 10
   Inheritance, 10, 13
   Juvenile onset, 27-34
   Longevity and, 145
   Nature of, 8
   Non-inherited forms of, 15
   Precipitating factors, 14
   Prevention of, 15
   Retinopathy, 128
   Symptoms, 10
   Time zone changes and
      meal times, 147
   Treatment of, 15
      Adult onset, 19-21
      Oral anti-diabetic treatment, 25, 82
      Responsibility of diabetic.
         In introduction, 4
      Use of other medicines, 24, 25
Diabetic Children's Summer Camps, 33
Diabetic diets, 36-80
   Calculated, 39, 46
   Exchange, 39, 67
Diabetic ketoacidosis (acidosis), 124-125
Definition, 124
   Causes, 124
   Diagnosis, 125
   Prevention, 125

Symptoms, 125
Diabetic Neuritis, 126
   Definition, 126
   Other forms, 126
   Painful neuritis, 126
   Painless neuritis, 126
Diabinese (Chlorpropamide), 23, 82, 100
Diet, 36-80
   Adult Onset DM, 21
   Alcohol, 78-79
      Calculation in diet, 79
      Problems, 78
   Calculated, 39, 46
   Characteristics of diabetic, 36-37
   Exchange, 39, 67
   Foods to be avoided, 41-42
   Guidelines for following, 37
   Illness and dietary modifications,
   Juvenile Onset, 29
   Kinds of foods to use or avoid, 116-120
   Low calorie, 42
   Supplements, 42
   Vegetarian diets, 76
Diuretics, 25
Driving and hypoglycemia, 106
Dymelor (Acetohexamide), 23, 82-83, 100

E

Employment, 20, 143
   Associated with a chronic health
      problem, 143
   Associated with adult onset
      diabetes, 20
Epinephrine, 25
Exercise—effect on management, 21
Fat, 39, 79
Federal Aviation Administration, 148
Feet, 120-122
   Athlete's foot, 122
   Care of, 121
Food values, 50
Fertility and d.m., 139-142
Forsham, Dr. Peter, 14

G

Gamble, Dr. D.R., 13
Glossary, 183
Glucagon, 13
Glucose, 8-14
    Appearance in urine, 108
    Normal blood levels, 9
    Tolerance test, 9
    Urine tests for, 108
    Use by the body, 8
Guillemin, Dr. Roger, 14

H

Health insurance, 144
Hyperlipidemias, 137-139
Hyperlipoproteinemias, 137-139
Hypoglycemia (low blood sugar
    reactions), 100
    Causes of and prevent, 83, 103
    Hypoglycemia and driver's license, 106
    Nature of, 100
    Treatment, 104-106
        Glucagon, 104-105
        How to treat, 104
        Instant glucose, 106
        When to treat, 104
    Types, signs and symptoms, 102
        Cerebral cortex effect, 102
        Epinephrine effect, 102

I

Instant glucose, 106
Insulin, 9, 10, 84-100
    Adjustment of insulin dose, 96-99
        Factors which lower blood
            sugar, 97
        Factors which raise blood
            sugar, 96
        Guidelines for adjustment
            of dose, 97, 99
        Insulin action curves, 98
    Administration of, 89-95
    Beta cells, 9
    Care of insulin when traveling, 99
    Equipment used for injection, 87, 88
    Facts about, 85
        Concentrations, 85
        Types, 87
        U-100, 84, 85, 86
    Hypoglycemia and, 100-107

    Local reactions from insulin
        injection, 94
        Bruises, 95
        Insulin allergy, 95
        Lipodystrophies, 94
    Preparation for home use, 87
        Care of equipment, 88
        Equipment, 87, 88
        Filling the syringe, 89, 90
        Injection, 89, 91, 92-93
        Selection of site, 90, 91
    Reactions to its use, local, 94
    Results of too little, 10
    Sites for injection, 91
    Use by the body, 9, 11
    Where produced, 9
Insurance for Diabetics, 144

J

Juvenile, or insulin-dependent
    diabetes mellitus,
    Characteristics, 27
    Children's camps, 33
    Control factors, 32
    Diet, 28-29
    Exercise—influence of, 30
    Insulin, 29
    Mental attitude, 30
    Objectives of treatment, 28
    Stress, 31
    Symptoms, 27
    Treatment, 28
        diet, 28
        Insulin, 29

K

Ketoacidosis (see diabetic
    ketoacidosis), 124-125
Ketostix—urine test for ketones, 113
Kidney infections, 127
Kipnis, Dr. D., 18

L

Laser, Argon, 130
Life Insurance, 144
Liver, 9
    Function in preventing
        low blood glucose, 101

Low blood sugar reactions, see
  hypoglycemia
Luft, Dr. R., 130

M

Machemer, Dr. R., 131
Meat, food values, 59, 72
Medical identification, see hypo-
  glycemia
Menstruation, 139

N

Najarian, Dr. J., 128
Neuritis—(see diabetic neuritis), 126
Nephropathy—diabetic, 127, 128

O

Obesity, 14, 134
  As a health hazard, 19
  Ideal weight, 134, 135
  Problems of, 23
  Related to adult onset diabetes, 17
  Treatment of, 24, 136
  Types of, 136
Oral agents, 25
  Alcohol and, 78
  Classes of, 82
  Dose, size tablets, 82
  Hypoglycemia, 83
  Hypoglycemia and other
    medications, 83-84
  Side effects, 83
  Warning, F.D.A., 23
Oral contraceptives,
Orinase—(Tolbutamide), 23, 82, 100

P

Patient,
  Emotional adjustments, 30, 31,
    84, 85
  Responsibility for care, 4
Pearson, Dr. O.H., 130
Poulsen, Dr. J., 130
Pregnancy, 141, 142
Protein, 46

R

Recipes, 152-173
Reference list, 180
Retinopathy, Diabetic, 129

S

Simpson, Dr. Nancy, 13
Siperstein, Dr. M., 20
Somatostatin, 14, 131
Somogyi Effect, 103
Stomach flu and care of diabetes, 115
Stress, 14
  Accidents, 14
  Effect on diabetes, 14
  Emotional, 14
  Illness, 14
  Pregnancy, 14
  Surgery, 14
Summer Camps for children, 33
Sulfonylurea Drugs, 82
Symptoms,
  Juvenile diabetes, 27
  Adult onset diabetes, 17
Syringes, 86, 87
  Care of, 88, 89
  Types, 87, 88

T

TesTape—urine test for glucose, 110
Tolazamide—(see Tolinase), 100
Tolinase (Tolazamide), 82-83, 100
Tolbutamide—(see Orinase), 100
Travel tips, 144
Treatment of diabetes mellitus, 15
  Adult onset d.m., 21
    Acute illness, treatment, 115, 116
    Diet, 21, 36, 46, 67, 116
    Exercise, 21
    Insulin, 84
    Oral agents, 23, 82-84
    Problems, 23
    Results, 24
  Juvenile onset d.m., 28-32
    Acute illness, treatment of, 115,
      116
    Attitude, 30
    Diet, 29, 36, 46, 67, 116
    Exercise, 30
    Insulin, 29, 84
    Results, 32
Patient responsibility, 4

U

Unger, Dr. Roger, 13
Urine glucose—cause, 10
Urine tests for glucose and
    ketones, 108, 111
  Drugs affecting urine tests, 110
  Reasons to test, 108
  Records of urine tests, 113, 114
  Tests for glucose, 108
    Clinitest, 109, 110
      5-drop method, 109
      2-drop method, 110
    Clinistix, 110
    Diastix, 110
    Testape, 110
  Tests for ketones (acetone), 112
    Acetest tablets, 112
    Ketodiastix, 113
    Ketostix, 113
  Time of testing, 111, 116
  24-hour collection, 111

V

Vegetables, food values, 50, 67
Vegetarian diets, 76

W

Visual disorders, 128-131
  Cataracts, 129
  Retinopathy, 129
    Development of, 129
    Hypophysectomy, 130
    Laser therapy, 130
Vitamins, 76, 77
Vitrectomy, 130, 131
Vitreous Hemorrhage, 130

W

Weight
  Ideal weight, 135
West, Dr. K., 14
White, Dr. P., 10
Williamson, Dr. J.R., 20

Y

Yalow, Dr. R., 18

Z

Zweng, Dr. C., 130

Cover and book design: Dean McMullen